WONDERFULLY WELL

HOW WE LOST 132 POUNDS AND HEALED OUR BODIES

PLUS

A COLLECTION OF WHOLE FOOD RECIPES AND MENUS FROM THE WELLNESS WORKSHOP

Psalm 139:14

I will praise You for I am fearfully and wonderfully made.

Marvelous are Your works and that my soul knows very well.

Celeste & Phil Davis

Food & Lifestyle Coaching

Wonderfully Well Publishing
Crescent, Oregon

Wonderfully Well

Copyright 2014 by Celeste & Phil Davis

Third Edition

We are not dieticians, nutritionists or medical professionals. We are food experts and lifestyle coaches who have experienced and live everything we teach. Our mission is to lead you toward developing a taste for many satisfying, real, whole, healthy foods. To some, a new food plan can seem overwhelming and time consuming, but we are here to help you shop, prep, plan, store, and serve excellent nutritious food. We would also love to help you set up your kitchen!

This book is not intended to diagnose, treat or offer medical advice of any kind. Information in this book is intended for educational purposes only. Please consult with a licensed medical professional for all matters concerning your health. You assume full responsibility for the use and practice of any material in this book and full liability for results.

The term "use" assumes, as an individual, you are taking full responsibility and liability for your health care and lifestyle decisions.

ISBN 978-0-578-06229-7
Printed in the United States of America
Wonderfully Well Publishing
PO Box 182
Crescent, Oregon 97733
615-975-0186   www.thewellnessworkshop.org

It is true God does everything Wonderfully Well, including the people He strategically places in our lives.

Our lives, our bodies, our minds and our gifts belong solely to Him and Him alone and we are thankful that when we call, he answers and does all things well.

IT IS HIM WE THANK FOR STRATEGIC PEOPLE IN OUR LIVES.

Our parents who raised us to walk in the wisdom and fear of The Lord.

Our marriage, orchestrated by our loving heavenly Father to provide encouragement and companionship as we walk this journey together.

Our children, Jesi and Robb and grandchildren, Josiah and Ian, whom we hope will be able to navigate a better life because of our journey.

Our extended family, friends and clients who have walked with us, encouraged us and joined us as we have become Wonderfully Well.

There are eight women we must acknowledge who contributed much time and energy to this and other projects. To them we are ever so grateful.

Janice Gietzen who told me for years "you should write a book", even before I had anything to write about and who rescued me from some formatting errors over her July Fourth holiday!

Michelle Mykeloff, my inspiration to create a truly professional product. Thank you Michelle for the hundreds of hours you spent pouring over my written materials for a future project, which to organize helped me to organize my thoughts in a way that will help others. Thank you to her daughters, Kayla, 10 and Alyssa, 13 (of course now they are growing up) for allowing me to "learn with them" as we cooked together and their willingness to try and learn to love new and healthier foods.

Kay York, our Whole Foods class "watch dog" who diligently reminds me of things I forget such as, "did you put the eggs in yet" or "should that come out of the oven now"? Thank you Kay for the many hours you spent going through every recipe with a fine toothcomb, for preparing our recipes for your friends and family and for helping to make them useable for other people.

Carol Johnson, a gifted creative editor who asked questions that caused me to dig deeper, explain better and hopefully inspire more. Thank you for working with our budget and using your gifts in a way that will help others on their journey.

Kristen Terry and her family for taking the book, reading it and going through the detox without coaching to make sure it would work and then giving me feedback to make it work! Thank you to her children, Jocelyn, 10 and Brendon, 9 for coaching your friends into healthy eating as well.

Sharon Taylor, our wonderful book cover and web designer. Thank you for the hundreds of hours you put in to make our cover and site Wonderfully Well. It is amazing how God prepared you for helping us by taking you on your own journey to health 13 years ago and how he put us together in such an unusual and yet divine way.

Thank you to the entire Priszner family, friendships restored after more than 20 years. Thank you Texanna for inspiring the family to do our program; for holding on to the belief for

82 years that the body needed to be cleansed and healed with good food and for persevering in our program even through your own physical difficulties.

Thank you Nancy (well, OK, Roy too) for becoming the "star student" as you have completely changed your recipes, pantry and your family's health for the better. Thank you for the extra effort you put towards good food for the handicapped people you care for and giving them a new measure of health and wellness. Thank you for being a cheerleader, promoter and sharing some of your recipes with us as well.

Thank you to my step-dad, Don Rutledge for detailing with me! You know what I mean.

There are seven medical professionals who impacted Celeste's view that good health is attainable. To them we are ever so grateful.

Thank you to Dr. Chris Edwardson, M.D. who trained Celeste in 1990 as a back office medical assistant. I clearly remember your words my first day "Most of our patients symptoms have emotional and spiritual roots", this gave me the first glimpse into true healing and opened many questions in my mind about the body, mind and spirit connection.

Thank you to Dr. Daniel Mc Cleary, D.C. who allowed Celeste to type his notes and learn the cause and effect of food and lifestyle on the human body. It is from you I learned about the body's ability to heal itself.

Thank you to Dr. Craig Roles, D.C., you were the one who pushed us into the deep end of becoming truly healthy. You were God's answer to my cry for help. Thank you for not letting me quit!

Thank you Dr. Michele Benoit for believing in Celeste, giving me a chance to start out, sharing your clinic, your patients, your knowledge and your life.

Thank you to Dr. Kathleen Inman, D.C. for putting your heart into your detox program with me what a blessing to see the amazing results in your personal life and for encouraging your patients to eat well.

Thank you to Dr. Gregory Skye for helping me to remember that my Abba Father is the one who always has my back and encouraging me to always seek His counsel in my life and work.

Thank you to Dr. Rowen S. Pfeifer, D.C. for attending almost every class we teach, being a devoted follower of Jesus and encouraging everyone about the importance of eating well for health.

There are hundreds of clients we must acknowledge who allowed us to share in their journey. It is ultimately because of our work with you that others will be helped through this book.

To you we are ever so grateful.

"We strongly endorse the lifestyle choices supported in this book. Celeste and Phil were "star pupils" in their quest for health when they first came to our clinic years ago. It was great to see their lives change in front of us. It is true that your life too can radically change when you learn the powers of purification and of committing to a healthy lifestyle.

The most common benefits we witness are significant long term weight loss, substantial gains in energy and deeper sleep. We have also seen surgeries avoided and chronic pain disappear. The body is quite amazing in its ability to heal when we feed it right and when we, more importantly stay away from the foods that are "slowly killing us".

We encourage you to take the next step and create a new life for yourself!"

Dr. Craig Roles, DABCI, DCBCN
Board Certified Chiropractic Internist and Clinical Nutritionist
Susie Roles
Wellness Coach/Yoga Pilates Certified Trainer
Green Valley Chiropractic and Wellness Center
Henderson, Nevada

"A Must-have for anyone wanting to transform their life by living healthier; body, mind and soul!"

Dr. Kathleen Inman, D.C.
Inman Chiropractic Health and Wellness Center
1302 Central Court
Hermitage, Tennessee 37076
615-414-7914
inmanchiro@gmail.com
http://inmanchiro.com

"Celeste's ideas compliment any chiropractic care, acupuncture, osteopathic or wellness practice. Total body modification cannot happen unless lifestyle is changed. The Wellness Workshop detox and healthy lifestyle program has allowed my patients to feel the difference in their pain (reduction) and be able to make the necessary changes.

As an applied kinesiologist, it truly has taught me the ability of raw foods to strengthen the body naturally. Our work with Celeste has been a valuable lesson for my patients but even more for me to achieve total wellness. Thank You Celeste!"

Dr. Michele Benoit, D.C.
Benoit Chiropractic and Wellness Center
321 Billingsly Court, Suite 10
Franklin, Tennessee 37067
615-261-3152
drmichelebenoit@yahoo.com
http://benoitchiropractic.com

"I have known Celeste and Phil Davis for a couple of years now and have attended many of their food preparation workshops at the Health food markets in Franklin, Tennessee. They have a large following every time they hold a class and their presentations are full of all the normal essentials as well as offering many useful hints and tidbits that make eating healthy more enjoyable and less work or time intensive. They have a fun and entertaining style that holds the attention of the crowd and the recipes are always great. I love to sample what they have prepared. In addition, they love the Lord and are truly ministering to the health needs of the people they serve. I highly recommend this book to anyone seeking healthy, fast and easy recipes to enhance the health of the entire family."

Dr. Rowen S. Pfeifer, DC
Living Health Chiropractic, Inc., Brentwood, TN
Health Minister for *Hallelujah Acres, Author of* **Healing God' Way**
615-714-1877

CONTENTS

NUTRITION KEY FOR RECIPES

GF   Gluten Free

DF   Dairy Free

SF   Sugar Free

NSO   Natural Sugar Only

HF   High Fiber

HP   High Protein

LF   Low Fat

BF   Beneficial Fats

NV Not Vegetarian

CHAPTER 1   OUR STORY

We were like everyone else, young, fit, and healthy and in love. Like many young people from the 1970's, Phil and I jumped into married life and started running full speed ahead. By the time we had been married 30 years we had almost doubled our marriage weight, Phil, going from 140 pounds at age 20 to 249 pounds at age 49. Celeste going from 120 pounds at age 18 to 240 pounds at age 47.

In addition to the excessive weight we were growing older with a plethora of health problems such as Type 2 Diabetes, Irritable Bowel Syndrome, Chronic Eczema, Plantar Fasciitis, back pain, addictions to alcohol and nicotine and male prostate problems. In just 4 months, after going through a body detoxification program and changing our eating and lifestyle habits, we lost a combined total of 132 pounds. We were amazed as our bodies healed from ALL of our medical problems and addictions. We maintain our good weight and health to this day.

FEARFULLY AND WONDERFULLY MADE

It is interesting to look back at life from 52 years of age, and realize we had everything we needed to maintain good weight and good health from our childhood. We were indeed, "fearfully and wonderfully made".

Phil is the middle child of four children. His family did not have a lot of refined and processed foods available until his teenage years. An athlete from a young age, Phil enjoyed physical challenges and knew how to push past his body's objections for a good workout. Phil was never one to sit around or be lazy.

Celeste's family changed to an extremely healthy diet when she was 13. Her mother, La Verne, was diagnosed with rheumatoid arthritis at just 31 years of age with 4 children to care for and another child on the way. Celeste's mother, at the encouragement of a friend, began following the advice of early nutrition advocate, Adele Davis, from the book <u>Let's Eat Right to Keep Fit</u>. La Verne began to quickly heal from her rheumatoid arthritis and enthusiastically fed her family good, whole foods. Treats changed from left over wedding cake and lumps of frosting every weekend to whole grain cookies and breads made with honey. This was my first opportunity to change.

This sudden change in food was drastic for me and my brothers and sisters who had previously enjoyed pieces of wedding cake for breakfast which were leftovers from our mother's catering business. Suddenly, it seemed, mother began feeding us stew for breakfast and making her own yogurt and bread. When we had tests at school she made "Tiger's Milk" to give us brain power, a shake consisting of orange juice, raw eggs, brewer's yeast and who knows what else. It tasted awful. To be honest, I did not see these changes as opportunity. In fact the changes made me angry and I determined when I was on my own I would eat what I wanted, when I wanted. No more of that awful health food for me! Little did I know these changes were actually God's gift to me, a way for me to avoid my genetic pre-disposition to Type 2 Diabetes and its associated maladies. While I knew this disease was in my heritage and possibly in my future, I decided to think about it when I was "old", perhaps before I turned 30.

OUR FORMER "FOOD LIFE"

The first time either of us ate pizza from a restaurant was on a group date with four other teenage couples, when I was 15 and Phil was 17. Our mothers had made homemade pizza growing up but we had never had the "real thing". We were both excited about the "Hula Lula" pizza; Canadian bacon with pineapple.

That night was a turning point in our lives, shortly after that group date we ditched the people we had been dating and fell head over heels in love with each other. It was also a point of addiction for me. I was hooked on eating out and quickly developed a taste for junk food. Our dating was often centered on food such as root beer floats at "A& W", "Burrito Supremes" (usually more than one) from Taco Bell a burgeoning West Coast franchise, or an occasional salad with our French Dip sandwiches and fries. Phil's salad request was always "drown it in blue cheese please; I want the lettuce coming up for the last time".

I worked as a kitchen aide and dishwasher at Dallas Care Center in Dallas, Oregon during my high school years. The kitchen was always full of desserts, cookies and soda pop, a true haven from what I considered to be my families "health food hell" at home. My boss, Jean Robertson, truly loved the teen-age workers she patiently trained. She was constantly yelling at me as I munched on another cookie, "you're going to get fat if you keep eating like that", of course, I thought she was crazy!

After our marriage, Phil lived on Mountain Dew and Doritos and still wanted his meat and potatoes after a hard day's work at the plywood mill in Dallas, Oregon. When I was pregnant with our first child, Jesi, my obstetrician told me I should walk every day. Phil and I enjoyed walking daily to the new Dairy Queen in town where I got my "calcium" from a Peanut Buster Parfait.

Recently we were on our six-mile walk and remembering our former "food life". One of the mileposts of success in our marriage was when we could afford a second refrigerator that was always stocked with a variety of soda pop, a freezer full of ice cream and a pantry full of chips and cookies. Of course the main refrigerator was for the health food; butter, cheese, lots of meat, various condiments and the occasional vegetables and fruits. We laugh at the irony that today we are thrilled to have a 25-pound bag of organic carrots, and a refrigerator full of fresh organic fruits and vegetables. Our new milepost of success is our well-used Champion juicer! Thank You God!

MISSED OPPORTUNITIES FOR HEALTHY CHANGE

After our daughter Jesi was born my grandmother invited me to join her at Weight Watchers. I now know my family was concerned about my steady weight gain. After Jesi's birth my weight went from 120 to about 160. I went to Weight Watchers a few times "for Grandma Toots" but didn't stick with it. No one ever said to me "Celeste, I am concerned about your weight gain. You are so beautiful and have such a lovely body, don't allow yourself to gain any more, let's work on this together." Maybe they were afraid of me, maybe they did say it, and I just didn't hear it. Regardless, these "back door" approaches did not work.

When our daughter Jesi was a toddler my parents introduced us to Shaklee, a health food and vitamin membership company. Phil and I started teaching "Shaklee Slim Clubs". We were very successful and enjoyed the relationships we made with people. The heads of our organization were sure we would become high producers and invested much time and money in our business. We saw this time in our lives as preparation for ministry, learning we were both quite good at teaching and speaking, and had a heart for bringing people to a personal relationship with Jesus Christ.

One day Phil came home and said, "I believe God is calling me to full time ministry, I need to be preaching Jesus instead of Shaklee". Consequently, we left our new "healthy life" and dove into full time pastoral ministry with all of its coffee meetings, pizza parties and church potlucks. That is when we really began to gain weight. I quickly packed on another 25 pounds in our first 3 years of ministry and Phil was frequently teased about going from a size 32 waist to a 36 waist by the time he was 30.

A few short years after our marriage, Phil's father had a severe heart attack caused by blockages and had bypass heart surgery. He made drastic changes to his diet and began a workout program. As of this writing he has outlived most of his peers and maintains good health for his age of 90 year.

There were many other times God brought opportunities for me to change and I did not receive them because of my rebellion. I was not going to let anyone control my food; therefore food began to control me.

Other missed opportunities included my good friend Katherine Olson who religiously followed the Fit for Life plan, and was in excellent shape even after the birth of three children. Then there were my fellow children's pastors and dear friends at Westside Church in Bend, Oregon, where I was the only staff member who was obese. Karen was a college level swimmer and fitness expert and Cynthia, a professional ski instructor and gymnast. These professionals had offered to work out with me and help me get in shape many times. However, at 200 pounds, I was too afraid and ashamed to accept these gracious opportunities so I began to try and do it myself. Unfortunately it was another nine years before I admitted to God "I need your help, I can't do this by myself, please send someone to help me".

God had given us both opportunities to change our eating and health habits and we chose what tasted good, was

Convenient, what everyone else ate and sometimes deliberately what was unhealthy, out of rebellion. We are fearfully and wonderfully made, and God's grace was there when I finally asked for His help, he took me back to the roots of my childhood, whole, natural, God-made foods. What about you?

Have *you* asked for and received God's help? This is an opportunity for you...take full advantage of this opportunity to Improve Your Health by Changing Your Food!

MY PEOPLE PERISH FOR LACK OF KNOWLEDGE.
HOSEA 2:4

Now that we have experienced good health and left behind our sedentary, fast food ways, we are passionate about sharing truth with those around us. In America, much of our life is spent talking with family, friends and acquaintances about health conditions, doctor's visits and aches and pains. We now know, according to a study done by the American Medical Association, that 98% of the physical and emotional conditions Americans experience are directly related to diet and lifestyle. Only 2% are attributed to genetics. Phil and I want people to know they don't have to be sick, weak and helpless as they grow old weak.

This book is a combination of our struggles, our victories, the plan we follow and the recipes we use. All of the recipes have been tested with our family and friends, clients, the patients of the doctors we have worked with and at our Health food market cooking classes over the past four years. The plans are provided as a start. As you add healthy foods to your life you will come up with your own favorite menu ideas and the alkaline food plan and detox plan will be your framework. This is the second cookbook I have written. The first one was for my daughter about 10 years ago; it included all of the recipes she loved growing up; some from me, some from grandma, aunts and many from the different churches where Phil used to work as pastor. To this day, the memories behind the recipes are as precious as the recipes themselves.

Our typical Saturday morning breakfast was "pankuken" which are German pancakes similar to crepes, smothered in butter and powdered sugar. Our children devoured those with a healthy glass of 2% milk loaded with chocolate syrup. Today we enjoy the Spelt "Buttermilk" Pancake recipe in chapter 16, with real maple syrup, sweet and satisfying and a little healthier and love fresh squeezed grapefruit juice with our pancakes.

Phil was pastor of a church on an Indian reservation, the Confederated Tribes of Siletz. A popular community event was our Indian Taco Fry. The Siletz women were masters at creating the taco shells with white flour, eggs, and yeast, deep fried into a puffy round and topped with meat, sour cream, cheese, beans and salsa with a little iceberg lettuce and tomato to make it look good! Indian Fry Bread Tacos are a tasty food indeed, but a heart attack waiting to happen. Today we enjoy the 3 Bean Tacos, in chapter 15 or West Coast Fish Tacos, in chapter 17. These new recipes are delicious and have very little saturated fat and lots of nutrition.

Our family always loved to go to the grandparent's house where there was never a shortage of treats. It was my goal to be just like Grandma Davis. She had a huge kitchen drawer FULL of a grand assortment of junk food such as Ding Dongs, Fritos, Sugar Cookies and the like. That drawer was accessible to all family members who were able to crawl and pull themselves up to the drawer, for most of the grandkids it was about age 10 months! Did I mention the freezer full of ice cream and the 2-liter bottles of soda lined up along the garage wall? Junk food heaven! We dreamed about Grandma Davis' Oatmeal Chocolate Chip Cookies loaded with canola oil, brown and white sugar, not to mention chocolate chips made with high fructose corn syrup. Now we enjoy the much healthier, but just as delicious, version of that recipe in chapter 16, using nutritious Spelt flour, raw local honey, coconut oil and low sugar Enjoy Life Chocolate Chips. Grandma Davis was an excellent cook and she put her heart into her cookies, however, at the time there was little education about unhealthy foods.

Last year I threw out almost all those old, family recipes because the ingredients and the way they were prepared actually damage and slow down the healing and cleansing of the body. We now make food choices based on how the food will fuel, build and cleanse. So, having changed our outlook on food, recipes laden with refined sugars and chemicals such as those found in boxed cake and pudding mixes. Old staples such as canned soups, and pre-packaged sauces and of course, hormone-induced or dehydrated dairy, products, became unattractive in light of our new food preferences and desire for good health.

During the last four plus years of learning to eat healthy, I have built a new repertoire of recipes. Today I choose food to fuel my body rather than to find comfort, feeding my emotions or centering relationships on food. I now look for memories in relationships and activities. I seek comfort from my relationship with God. My emotions are more often positive because I lovingly speak my mind rather than stuffing my face with food. I learned that speaking my mind gives the same satisfaction I once received from eating, but with benefit to my body rather than harm. I have learned to use my voice and speak when necessary, seasoned with love and kindness, but always true to God and myself. My life today is more peaceful, even amid difficult circumstances, than it has been in my entire adult life.

HOW OUR CHANGE BEGAN

In 2004, I weighed 240 pounds and Phil, weighed 249 pounds. In addition to Type 2 diabetes, I suffered from frequent bouts of Irritable Bowel Syndrome (IBS), chronic eczema, Rosacea, Plantar fasciitis, mood swings, and depression.

Phil's health problems sounded like a typical drug advertisement for men and included low back pain, prostate issues with frequent yet difficult urination and male E.D. in addition to alcohol and nicotine addictions.

Looking back, our health issues were not so different from our friends and family. It seemed most people "our age" (I was 47; Phil 49) were beginning to break down physically in one way or another. I have a family history of diabetes, IBS, Rosacea and depression, so suffering from these diseases and other discomforts just appeared to be my lot in life, or so I had resigned to believe. I simply had to bear up under what I (falsely) considered part of the natural aging process.

I was diagnosed with Type 2 diabetes in 2000, just four years before Phil and I decided to try our first "whole foods" detox. I was 42 years old when I got the diagnosis and luckily that report pushed me to participate in a workplace wellness program with my employer. This program involved undergoing multiple tests including blood panels, blood pressure, weight, and body fat percentages; it also took into account family history and lifestyle practices to achieve what they called your "True Body Age". Upon completing a series

23

of various tests, my "True Body Age" at age 42 came back assessed as that of a 67-year old woman! I was shocked, horrified and scared. I decided to get on top of things physically. Even then, something told me I needed to eat a more natural diet. I started eating mostly unprocessed, home cooked meals and exercising. I did well, even dropped a few pounds. However, I certainly didn't' want to become a "crazy health food nut" and when our friend Jimmy Gietzen would suggest we go to Wild Oats Market, I quickly declined. Within a few months, I was back to my old ways and the weight came back plus more. Over the next 4 years, I tried many food plans until finally in January 2004, my weight at its highest, I became very ill with a respiratory infection that hung on despite antibiotics and different medications, until April of 2004.

In the fall of 2004, I was desperate, and I cried out to the Lord, "I need your help, I can't keep gaining weight. 250 pounds. is not very far away." That same year my husband and I made a major life change. We quit our jobs, sold our home and moved to Las Vegas (no, not to become professional gamblers), to be near our daughter and grandson. The physical move initiated a chain of events that would be the most positive change in my entire life; the life I live today is completely different than how I lived most of my adult life. Today I get excited about going for walks, creating new healthy foods, growing a garden and encouraging others towards their best life.

In August 2005, the answer to my cry for help came through finding a detox program that would change my thinking about food and life and inspire me to "improve my life by changing my food".

My new employer was Dr. Craig Roles, DC, DABCI, DCBCN, a chiropractor, and nutrition and detoxification specialist. I started working for him as a receptionist and consequently had a great deal of patient interaction. Often patients felt more comfortable sharing their challenges and even failures with me than the doctor because they didn't want to disappoint him or appear weak. I was responsible for helping them purchase supplements, took their questions over the phone and in general became a cheerleader. Dr. Roles asked me to try out his detox program so that I could better understand what his patients went through as they were coping with lifestyles changes. I reluctantly agreed and my husband Phil graciously agreed to join me. I am grateful to God for my husband's support as I see now this was all God's mercy and love to help me get rid of my unhealthy self.

21 days into an all-vegetarian detoxification program, I had lost 16 pounds, and my husband Phil had lost 21. Likewise, we had lost ALL (yes, ALL!) of our medical symptoms and conditions. My blood sugar counts had returned to normal (without the use of medication), and the IBS, eczema, Rosacea, depression, back pain, prostate issues, and male E.D. had disappeared! Within four months, Phil was also completely free of alcohol and after two more years he was able to completely kick nicotine dependencies.

WE BOTH FELT REVOLUTIONIZED!

Within days the painful eczema on my hands was gone and by the end of the 21 days my hands had a baby-fresh beautiful layer of new skin. My blood sugar stabilized within about three days and so my depression lifted, no more mood swings! Phil and I were both surprised how quickly our Irritable Bowel Syndrome went away making our elimination a blessing instead of a painful curse. It was in the detox period that Phil shared with me how devastated his prostate problems were and how elated he was when they too disappeared. We both experienced more energy, clearer thinking and felt much happier inside. It was amazing and puzzling to think all these wonderful things happened just by changing our food. Today the slogan of our business is "Improve Your Life by Changing Your Food.

There were other health modalities that sped our recovery. We both received chiropractic adjustments to help our nervous system recover. This was a vital part of our healing. We walked at least 30 minutes per day. Celeste also had a different form of massage each week and eventually, a total of 36 colon hydrotherapy sessions. One of the programs our clients can choose from is called the Total Health Makeover and includes all four of the natural healing modalities that were a part of our healing. See chapter 19 for more information on these modalities and check our website for practitioners in your area.

We began to walk every day, an important part of restoring our health. We started out by walking in the evenings after our protein shake and veggies; we walked about 30 minutes a day. Over the years we began to increase our distance. Today we walk more than 6 miles almost every day and run anywhere from 1 to 4miles.

HOW WE CONTINUE TO LIVE WELL

Our bodies, minds, and spirits felt so great after those first 21 days, why would we go back to our old ways? So, we continued to eat according to the "wellness" program that Dr. Roles had introduced to us. Over the next 4 months we lost a combined total of 132 pounds. We have a personal commitment to good health body, mind and spirit and rely on God to maintain these good changes to this day.

Every aspect of our physical health improved and we began an exercise program of walking and running almost every day. Today we walk and run a total of 6 miles almost every day. We look and feel much younger than our current ages of 52 and 54. Phil had a "middle age" physical at the beginning of this year. The doctor was amazed at how strong and healthy Phil is. After his examination, Phil's doctor said, "when you are healthy at 14 years of age it is genetic but when you are healthy at 54 years of age it is all about the choices you make." He congratulated Phil for his good choices and told him he is in excellent health.

At age 51, I took the "True Body Age" test again, just to see what my stats would be, and just 4 years after changing my diet and lifestyle, the test revealed my "True Body Age" was actually comparable to a woman of 42! Amazing, even though 9 years had passed since the first time I took that test, my body was acting, looking, and feeling as if I were 42 again! I truly felt I had regained those years that were lost...remembering that at the actual age of 42 and the time of my first test, the "True Body Age" my body reflected was 67. With the second test results, I had become 9 years younger and healthier. When God does something, He does it well; we truly ARE fearfully and wonderfully made.

WHAT WE EXPERIENCED DURING OUR DETOX

I cannot say our life transition has been easy, but it has definitely been simple; simple in thought and practice. We've learned to eat real whole foods, as close to the natural state as possible. Non-processed fruits and vegetables, limit the amounts of animal protein we intake (meat, fish, chicken, turkey, eggs, cheese, yogurt, milk) and add more plant protein to our diet. Simple. But totally opposite of everything I had been taught and practiced my entire life.

I've learned through this process that God seems to challenge our belief system and initiate positive change. His ways are usually simple in practice; however so different from the ways of man, they sometimes seem drastic. The simplicity of our new lifestyle is reflected in our choices. Fresh fruits and vegetables make up the largest portion of our food; really not too difficult to think about.

In the first 3-5 days of our initial detox we still craved our pizza, sodas and comfort foods. We experienced withdrawal from coffee, sugar and fatty foods. It seemed like it took much longer to prepare the good foods and to be honest, at first they didn't taste so great. However, it was our experience and many others report the same experience, once we were off the addictive chemicals in processed foods, once we had cleared our bodies of caffeine and sugar, we no longer craved foods we had eaten too much of for years!

Before our detox Phil lived on Mountain Dew, Doritos and ice cream. I ate at least one chocolate cake donut every day and designer coffees several times a week. We ate out frequently and our food at home was based around meat and potatoes or bread and cheese. I am very sorry to say that we raised our children to be junk food junkies, our favorite family night for most of their lives was what we called "Davis Binge Night", how awful is that? How about "Davis Let's-Get-Drunk-On-Sugar-And-Fat" night? The entire family would take a trip to the grocery and everyone could pick out whatever junk they wanted to eat and they didn't have to share it with anyone else if they didn't want to.

Now we crave fresh squeezed grapefruit juice as a treat and prefer a vegetable soup to a roast beef dinner. We laugh as we eat sometimes, realizing we would have never chosen this way of life and now we would never give it up. So prepare yourself because this food plan is counter-American culture and even counter-church culture according to some of the places of worship Phil and I have belonged during parts of our lives.

Phil and I are passionate about the simple truths we have learned. We try to encourage everyone we meet, "<u>you don't have to grow old and be weak and sick</u>", a truth proven by thousands who change to a whole foods diet. Many people want to believe this truth but find it hard to believe good health could be true for them personally. There are many people who want to be sick, they prefer to go to a doctor and get pills and never get well. The media loudly proclaims the virtues (except for the minor side effects like "suicidal tendencies or heart failure") of the latest drug that will solve all our health problems, knowing that the drug they currently take hasn't helped at all. Changing to a healthy lifestyle is much more cost effective than losing weeks or months of work due to surgeries, doctor's visits and sick days. It is also much more fun. The change, however, can be scary and learning the truth can be time consuming.

We hope this cookbook takes you easily step-by-step through a great transition in your life! The book is designed to be more than a mere cookbook. We want it to be a manual to a life-long lasting change, showing you everything you may want to change from the kitchen equipment, to the staple products to keep in your pantry. By sharing our experience and research, you can achieve success.

This book contains weekly food plans along with some company and holiday menus. You will eventually develop your own style, your own favorites and your own convictions based on how your body reacts to food.

I sincerely hope this cookbook will make your journey easier. Everything in this book we learned the hard way. We spent HOURS researching, reading, experimenting, teaching and learning from others. It has taken approximately 2000 hours of educating ourselves to learn the information in this cookbook. The things we learned improved our life and the lives of our entire family. We know this can improve your loved one's lives too.

Give Your Body a Break from digestion by eating easy to digest foods.

Give Your Body a Break from toxins by eating organic and unprocessed foods.

Give Your Body a Break from toxic lifestyle habits by eating nutritious foods that helps the mind and emotions to work correctly.

Give Your Body a Break from toxic thoughts by learning to walk in forgiveness rather than resentment and bitterness.

Give Your Body a Break from negativity by practicing a thankful and grateful heart.

CHAPTER 2   THE DETOX MIRACLE

In just 28-days our bodies healed from type 2 diabetes, irritable bowel syndrome, chronic eczema (my hands were completely broken out all the time to the point of bleeding), plantar fasciitis (your heels hurt when you walk), depression, low back pain, male prostate issues without drugs or medical treatments.

WHY DID THIS PROGRAM WORK WHEN OTHERS FAILED

I tried many different diets over the years. Shaklee Slim Plan, Weight Watchers, South Beach Diet, Atkins, Fasting (aka: Starvation) and none of them produced lasting results. I would lose a few pounds and gain back more. Currently Phil and I are in our fifth year of maintaining the weight we lost and the good health we gained.

Everything was different in our detox program. First, we drank water like crazy, half our body weight in ounces. Later I learned that it takes three molecules of water to whisk away one molecule of fat. At 240 pounds, half our body weight in ounces was a lot of molecules of water!

I think our beverage consumption was the biggest change. We stopped drinking caffeinated drinks, sodas and using any form of sugar or non-sugar sweetener. This helped our bodies to let go of inflammation.

The final big change was eating real, unprocessed foods, as close to nature as possible. The only thing we monitored (no calorie counting) was twice as many veggies as fruits, that's it!

Our only fat was from vegetables, fruits and a little fat in our salad dressings, our only sugar was from vegetables and fruits. We had no grains whatsoever. We lost weight and began to feel GREAT!

Prior to undergoing a detox program, all of my attempts at restoring my health were based on the medical model of disease; disease management. Natural health realizes that the body is created to heal itself. Natural and ancient health practices focus on removing things that may inhibit good body function and then giving the body the fuel and building materials it needs to do its job correctly. I found that when I removed the foods that were "offending" my body and started eating the foods that gave my body what it needed to rebuild stronger, my body healed itself very quickly. Today, when I eat something that offends my body, I know it very quickly, usually within about 10 minutes. Once that food is eliminated, my body goes to work repairing and restoring good function.

For instance, coffee is something we consider a treat, we only have it occasionally, we only have really good coffee and I enjoy it with organic cream. If I drink coffee one day; I have no problem. If I drink coffee two days in a row, the third day I wake up feeling hung over. The cream and coffee are offending foods to my body, due to the addictive qualities of the caffeine and the body's inability to digest dairy products. The hung over feeling makes me crave coffee, which is something I never do, unless I drink it twice in a row! My remedy? I drink coffee less than one time a week.

We love feeling great! This is the basis for both Phil and I staying on track with our eating. We carefully weigh decisions to eat celebration foods, much like one checks their bank account before spending large amounts of money; can we afford to not feel good, will the pleasure of the food be worth it? Sometimes the answer is YES! Let's Celebrate! We take extra digestive enzymes and get out and walk the next morning to walk off the "bad food hangover". Many times on our up to 6-mile (or sometimes 10 mile) walks we thank the Lord, literally, that we can get out there and walk that far at our age. We are in this place because of God's answer to prayer.

Before starting our detox program, our clients take a detox questionnaire that shows the relationship to foods and the way they feel physically. In the first week most people see a 50% reduction in their physical complaints and up to100% of their complaints are gone in just 28-days. Why? Because they remove the offending foods and give their body what it needs to function properly.

WHAT TOXINS ARE PRESENT IN YOUR LIFE

Give Your Body a Break **from potentially toxic supplements and drugs.** Occasionally clients who are taking nutritional supplements or pharmaceutical drugs find those supplements and drugs are offending their bodies rather than helping them. You can check your medications for "rare" side effects on the website www.rxlist.com.

Seek help from a nutrition professional for advice on supplementation. Dr. Rowen Pfeifer *warns "supplements are to <u>supplement and not replace</u> a healthy diet and lifestyle. Use whole, mostly raw food and healthy life habits to achieve good health and supplements to fill in the gaps."*

Never take yourself off the medications your doctor prescribes for you, but do your homework and know what you are taking, use a compounding pharmacy who really cares about you, go to the same pharmacy all the time and ask their input about the drugs and symptoms you are experiencing. Always communicate with your doctor about your findings before stopping medications as many of them have serious side effects if you stop them immediately; in the drug world they call it "withdrawal". Some doctors don't know much about nutrition and others are really into it. Ask your doctor what their nutrition education and philosophy is. To find a well-balanced medical doctor go to http://restorativemedicine.org/.

Give Your Body A Break **With Real Food.** Detox your body, begin to give it the fuel it needs and your doctor may start taking you off your medications because your blood pressure will be normal, your blood sugar will be normal, your cholesterol and triglycerides will be perfect and you will feel better than you have in years!

YOU CAN AGE WITHOUT FALLING APART

It is amazing how many people think that after 30 you start falling apart. That is NOT God's plan; it is something we have been conditioned to believe by our culture. At this writing I am 52 years old and my husband is 54. We get up with energy, ready for our day. We do not have any aches and pains, we sleep well, our food digests, we have great physical intimacy and we don't have brain fog or memory lapses. We feel as good as, or better, than we did in our twenties.

The Old Testament in the Bible tells of great men like Moses, Joshua and Caleb who lived strong until their death. Moses began to lead his people at the age of 40 and died at 120, the Bible says he was as strong at his death as he had been his entire life. Caleb and Joshua went in and conquered the enemy and took possession of the land God had given them at 85; they certainly were not feeble and weak.

34

Modern men also accomplish this health and strength in their senior years. Jack La Lane lived strong into his 90's. Norman Walker, an early healthy eating advocate and the father of modern juicing, lived strong into his hundreds after being told he was dying at age 55. George Malkamus, founder of Hallelujah Acres, is in his 70's and living strong after allowing his body to heal naturally from cancer over 30 years ago. In fact, in 2008 we heard him tell the story of going for his "senior citizen" driver's license renewal. After the required vision test he was told he no longer needed to wear the glasses he had worn for most of his adult life, his vision was now normal! Reverend Malkamus is a living tribute to the wonders of 30 + years of daily carrot juice.

God is ultimately in control of the length of our days. We all know of people, (however I believe they are relatively few), through whom God chooses to reveal his glory through sickness, accidents, even premature death.

We cannot control how long our lives are, but we CAN control and are actually held responsible to control how we handle the body God has given us. We are told in the New Testament, that our body is His Temple. As stewards of His Temple we need to give our body what it needs to function properly, so we can accomplish what He intended for us to accomplish.

WHAT DOES YOUR BODY NEED?

Give Your Body A Break **With Proper Rest.** You may have heard the saying "If the devil can't make you bad, he'll make you busy". That is true; if we are overextended in our time we can't take advantage of God's divine appointments in our day-to-day lives. If we are overextended on our time we will not have time to take care of our body, His Temple.

Many people tell me they are too busy to be healthy and yet as they age and go on one, two, three, five pharmaceutical drugs they begin to spend all their time and money on drugs and doctors. Doesn't it make more sense to arrange your schedule so you spend a few hours a week preparing and eating real food, getting some movement and proper rest rather than ending up spending HOURS each week in a doctor's office and the rest of your time recovering from procedures, surgeries and drugs?

This program works because it helps restore your body to its natural, healthy function. Your body was created to remove toxins (detox) on a daily basis. We assist the body in that process by getting proper amounts of rest, filtered water, movement, sunshine and by giving the body the nutrients it needs to do its job. In 1989 the American Cancer Research Center discovered the body cannot do its job of cleansing (detoxing) on a daily basis without fruits and vegetables, so if you aren't eating fruits and vegetables, you are toxic.

Your body was also created to rebuild stronger, not weaker, however, if your body is overloaded with toxins, it is unable to do the important functions, healing and rebuilding strong cells. When a cell dies, it creates an exact replica of itself. If the dying cell is full of toxic waste and weakened, the new cell will be full of toxic waste and weakened. If the dying cell is cleansed and fortified with vitamins and minerals, the new cell will be strong. Keep up that process and over time your body will be younger and stronger instead of weaker and sicker.

EFFECTIVE BODY DETOXIFICATION PROGRAMS

Remove the toxins. The worst toxins are in your food and your thoughts. Eat real, whole foods and practice gratitude.

Restore an alkaline balance. Damage and degeneration is caused by acid conditions in the body. The Give Your Body a Break Detox and the Detox, Etc life plan are food plans that alkalize the body.

Replenish nutrients. Eating a diet high in fresh fruits and vegetables is the best way to give your body the building materials it needs to cleanse, heal and rebuild strong.

Renew the body. When toxins are removed and nutrients are supplied the body begins to renew itself stronger. You have a new lining in your colon every three days, new skin every 28 days, new blood every 120 days, new organs every 7 years and a new skeletal system every 15 years.

When you give your body the proper building materials, those new body parts are stronger than the old ones. This is why someone like Jack La Lane who ate a nutrient dense, mostly fruit and veggie diet, is living strong into his 90's. The best tool to renew your body stronger is fresh vegetable and fruit juices.

WE BENEFIT FROM DETOXING IN OTHER WAYS

A natural progression in detoxing your body is change in other areas. As humans we want to operate from the process of feeling like changing, then thinking about it and then doing it. When we operate that way, we go back to our old ways quickly.

Phil & I both have experienced cleansing and purification of our hearts and minds as we detox our bodies. On my 10th day I became very emotional; people would look at me and I would cry. I asked Dr. Roles about this and his answer was, "you're detoxing, you'll get better"!

Over the years I've experienced other times of emotional detoxing and am not only stronger physically but emotionally and spiritually as well. Phil had begun to drink alcohol a number of years prior to our detox and it had become too much. The physical and emotional strength and mental clarity he achieved from cleansing his body filtered into other areas and by the time our 4 months of weight loss had passed, he stopped drinking alcohol permanently.

A profound principle states "Right Action brings Right Thinking". When you detox, you intentionally make a change, Right Action – eating real food. As you continue with that intention, you start thinking clearly, no more brain fog, more energy and new excitement for your future. Suddenly you realize you feel better! This helps you to stay on track.

This happens, not only in our lives, but also in the lives of our clients. As people begin to eat real food, they feel good and start to make great choices in other areas. Many become free from bitterness, resentment, unforgiveness and addictions. They start to live a life they choose, rather than being "drug" through life. They find new intention to accomplish the things they love. Intention brings confidence and a life of renewed purpose. Most importantly, most of our clients establish a newer, deeper relationship with God. They leave behind toxic habits, toxic thought patterns and begin walking in newness body, mind and spirit.

It's fun and rewarding to get emails and calls from various clients weeks, months and years later telling of the positive changes they have made in every part of their lives. Simple things like organizing their homes or starting an exercise program. Ending toxic relationships, reconnecting with the love of their lives or engaging in work or activities they love and thought they would never do, restoring relationships. Most importantly; reconnecting with God through a personal relationship with Jesus Christ and genuinely experiencing God's delight towards them as an individual.

Addressing heart issues is a huge part of the detoxing process. Most of us know when we have a heart that is full of toxic bitterness. We feel consumed with negativity and we realize our heart is locked up and we are unable to love others. As your body heals, your heart and mind will follow. Put aside fear and take advantage of the opportunity to heal your heart, seek out help if you can't do it alone. "Freedom in Christ Ministries" website has contact information for counselors who can help you with these issues.

Begin to receive forgiveness from God and extend forgiveness to others, first for the big things and then let it sink down into your everyday life. After your heart has dealt with forgiveness for the "big things," you'll be surprised how forgiving smaller things in life becomes easier, such as forgiving the person who pulls out in front of you on the highway, or the person who pushes angrily ahead in line. (Hence, some wonderful freedom . . . !) Forgiving yourself is one of the most important things you can do. Many people do not feel they can forgive themselves for things that happened decades before. Stacie Halprin is a woman who lost 350 pounds; she started her weight loss journey at over 500 pounds. Can you imagine the determination that took? In her book, Winning After Losing, Warner Wellness Publishing, she states

"Turning pain into power means making peace with things you honestly cannot change. If you continue to harbor grief, regret and disappointment over these things, you can lose sight of all the positive changes you have made."

Your job is to accept Christ's forgiveness for you, when you do that, you can let go of the things you hold against yourself and others. "He who is forgiven much forgives much." Jesus suffered the pain and rejection of sin so that we don't have to.

39

For some, even after accepting Christ's sacrifice as payment for our sin and forgiving ourselves, we still have baggage and hardship related to our old way of life. It is common for our wrong choices or things done against us by others to cause great loss. God said in Joel 2: 25-27 that He will restore the YEARS we have lost and we do not have to live in shame. He tells us we will eat in plenty and by SATISFIED and know that He is our God.

Accept Christ's sacrifice on the cross for your sin, and then ask God to restore the years of loss in your life and begin to watch Him do it! A great place for more information on this subject is www.needhim.org. Feel free to send us an email and we will be happy to pray with you.

Many natural health practitioners guide their clients into heart cleansing through practices such as yoga, meditation, eastern religious practices. These things may help to disconnect the worry for a time but if the heart is not changed, confusion begins to rule. If you have been involved in these things and find that your life is marked with confusion, that you are not able to rise above certain issues in your life, I encourage you to seek a personal relationship with the Creator of the Universe, God the Father and His son, Jesus Christ. Not another religion but a personal relationship. If you would like to understand more about what that means, visit the website, www.needhim.org.

Research has shown that people experience greater and more lasting change in working with a life coach. The biggest value of working with a life coach is the ability to work through these and other life issues with someone who is on your side. A frequent comment of our detox clients is *"turns out it really wasn't about the food at all"*. People see God do some amazing things as they participate with Him to cleanse their hearts as they cleanse their bodies. For more information on our coaching services, go to our website, www.thewellnessworkshop.org.

In Their Own Words:

"We have good news and bad news: the good news is we know why you're feeling sick. The bad news is that you are allergic to all foods but rice and barley."

Thus began my journey to health in 1995, when "What can I eat?" became my life's obsession. Chronic sinusitis, yeast infections, digestive problems and psoriasis plagued me.

Years of chemical treatments for the psoriasis left me with severe allergic reactions to medications and antibiotics. I found relief through acupuncture, regular chiropractic adjustments and supplements.

But the greatest life-changing improvements came when my chiropractor introduced me to Celeste Davis. Celeste's gentle coaching, along with her vast knowledge of nutrition, the human body and the human spirit, changed my life forever.

The detox diet was a chance to rest from the toxins I was unknowingly putting into my body day after day. After eliminating wheat, corn, dairy and sugar and following the diet and recipes recommended by Celeste, I lost 15 pounds, reduced the frequency of sinus and yeast infections, and the psoriasis lesions cleared. I recommend this detox diet for anyone who wants to take charge of their own well-being once and for all! LC, F,50+

Detoxing your body is a really good idea, however, if you are not able or ready to do a full detox program, you can just start eating well and the best way to eat well is to eat the food God made for people!

The Detox Miracle!

Improve Your Life by Changing Your Food!

Celeste at 240 lbs.   Phil at 249 lbs.

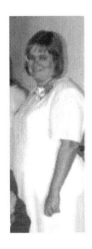 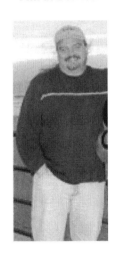

Lost in 21-days!

Celeste: Type 2 Diabetes, IBS, eczema, plantar fasciitis, back pain, achiness, mood swings.

Phil: Low back pain, frequent & urgent urination, prostate problems, male E.D., mood swings, dandruff.

Found in 21-days! Energy, freedom, new vision, joy. & Health!

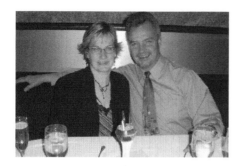

2005 4 months after our detox, continuing to eat well,

Celeste 176 lbs, ...Phil 193 lbs..............132 pounds removed!

No more illness!

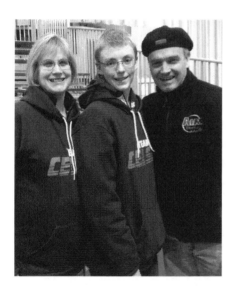

2014 We are at the Olympic Speed Skating Trials in Salt Lake City supporting JR Celski with our grandson, Josiah, 13. Josiah was the reason Celeste wanted to be healthy. Thankful.

CHAPTER 3   EAT PEOPLE FOOD

For centuries, people have eaten "people" food. What did they eat, you ask? Humans have cultivated foods from the ground, and used the animals that roamed their fields either to work as "cultivating machines" or become a consumable part of their food system. Historically, human food did not have any special dyes or colors, preservatives or additives until the early part of the Twentieth Century. Our great grandparents foods rotted quickly and much of the food could be eaten with little or no preparation.

Good nutrition for people is not that hard. You don't have to be a rocket scientist or a registered dietician to understand what people need to eat. God said it in the first chapter of the Bible in Genesis 1:29,

"See, I have given you every herb that yields seed which is on the face of all the earth, and every tree whose fruit yields seed; to you it shall be for food."

People food. Later in biblical history, after the great flood, God told Noah in Genesis 9:3,

"Every moving thing that lives shall be food for you. I have given you all things, even as the green herbs."

I don't see any mention of processed, chemical laden foods, do you?

The Standard American Diet Is Not True "People Food". Many Americans also wrongly assume the FDA (Food and Drug Administration) is protecting citizens from harmful foods. The truth is; the burden of proof is on the company producing the food. The FDA either accepts the data a company submits or rejects it; this is where money tends to talk louder than science. Companies hire specialists to perform "studies on a food to determine safety. These specialists are not hired by the FDA or an independent agency but by the food manufacturer who wants their product to pass. The "studies" are designed to produce the result the manufacturer desires. Dr. Joseph Mercola, MD, in his book <u>Sweet Deception</u> gives a perfect example of this type of "food safety study" on the product Splenda.

How big of a study would you expect to be done on a chemical sweetener that will be consumed by people from infancy throughout their lives? What types of data would be important to know if this chemical was safe? I am not a scientist, however, as a consumer I would want to know about long-term health effects, such as does it cause cancer? I would also be interested in the effect on hormone and brain function; will this chemical have any negative effects on those vital body systems? Also, how many people should be tested? When I ask this question to groups most people agree the number of people tested should be in the thousands, after all billions will be consuming these products.

Dr. Joseph Mercola revealed that the "studies" done to prove Splenda was not harmful were much less extensive than you and I would expect. In fact, Splenda was only tested on 36 people before being released for human consumption. Further, the testing was only done for 4 days to determine if it would cause cavities. Forgive my angst but come on, how can you tell if anything will cause cavities in just four days? Once again, I must emphasize, you are a steward of your body. You are responsible for your health; don't delegate that responsibility to your physician, the government, or your spouse.

Food expert, Michael Pollan, wrote a book called The Eaters Manifesto, asserting that basically there are three simple rules to healthy eating:

Eat Food (real food)   Mostly (raw) Plants   Not too much"

To Mr. Pollan's list I would add one more suggestion:

> Drink Filtered water, at least half your body weight in ounces every day.

If you follow these *four* guidelines for eating and hydrating your body, your health will improve, regardless of your age.

Phil's and my parents are still living vibrantly and have adopted some of the same eating habits we now encourage others to have.   Phil's father, Al, 89 at this writing swims several times a week and Al and Marylou, 80 enjoy walks in their neighborhood. Al made some serious changes to his eating habits after his bypass surgery when he was in his fifties.

Celeste's father, Stann leads a weight loss group in his hometown. He experienced great weight loss after going on the *Give Your Body a* Break detox at the age of 69. He was able to reduce his insulin by 60% and lost approximately 70 pounds over a two year period. Our family says he looks and even "sounds" better than we knew him for most of our adult lives.

Our parents continue to maintain better health than many of the people their age. Celeste's mother, LaVerne, called recently to report how much better she feels on this "real food" plan. At 71 years old, she began to really notice a physical deterioration throughout her entire body, to the point she was having extreme difficulty walking. After two months of eating a "real" food diet reported she is now going to a swimming class three days a week and last week end she mowed the lawn, fertilized the shrubs, cleaned off the deck and washed the windows in the back of her home. "I thought, man, this new way of life is making me stronger than I've been in years!"

This cookbook is designed to help you and your family transition to eating a healthier, life-giving food plan. Trust me, this change like all others is a process, but if you follow this nutritional advice, you will see a living revolution take place in terms of your health. Following are a few quick lists to give you a picture of what eating a real, "people food", "living diet" looks like.

WHAT WE EAT

Beverages

Purified spring water
Freshly made vegetable and fruit juices
Green tea and herbal teas

Foods

Fresh fruit
Mostly raw vegetables and a few cooked ones
Cooked beans almost every day
Eggs and cheese occasionally (less than 2 times per week)

Sprouted grain breads
Sprouted nuts and seeds

Condiments and Seasonings

Local raw honey, Stevia, raw Coconut sugar
Medjool dates instead of brown sugar
Celtic Sea Salt and freshly ground white pepper instead of black pepper
Fresh herbs and dried herbs for seasonings
Real organic butter or a healthy butter substitute called Earth Balance
Grape seed Veganaise or homemade mayonnaise instead of commercial mayonnaise

WHAT WE DON'T EAT

Some foods we consider "offending foods" because they are hard on our bodies, they don't digest well and produce inflammation. Therefore, we try to limit our consumption of this kind of intake. When we eat foods made with high fructose corn syrup and chemicals, or sugar or caffeine laden foods, we feel less energetic, the dull-minded-achy-body that was normal for most of our adult lives returns and we lose our edge. Everyone who begins to eat well finds their own level of comfort with these changes. The longer we eat well, the less we need or desire "treat" foods. The main treat for us is feeling great. When we do eat pizza, rich desserts or an occasional cup of coffee treats, we enjoy them once and then go back to our good, real people foods. At the end of this list is an explanation of how these foods may offend the human body.

Alcohol. This is a personal preference. We do not consume any alcohol.

Caffeine. This is a celebration food. Every once in a while (less than twice a month) we have a cup of coffee as a treat.

<u>Chemicals.</u> The only time we get chemicals in our food is when we eat out. We especially avoid MSG, artificial sweeteners and trans-Fats.

<u>Dairy.</u> We use raw cheese rarely. We go through approximately 8 oz. per month. We previously consumed about 5 pounds per week. We do not use cow's milk and only use cream in our rare cups of coffee.

<u>Meat.</u> This is like caffeine. I can count on two hands the times I have had meat in the last year. When we do eat meat we try to choose free-range chicken, grass fed beef and wild caught fish.

<u>Refined flour products</u> like bread, crackers, cookies, etc. We rarely eat bread other than Ezekiel or spelt bread.

<u>Sugar</u> in any form. If we eat refined sugar it is when we are away from home and involved in very rare and special occasions. Sugar includes brown sugar, white sugar, refined cane sugar, cane juice, organic sugar, beet juice, and of course the horrible "high fructose corn syrup". We NEVER use any artificial chemical sweeteners or Stevia combined with sugar. Our sweets come from honey, coconut sugar, Stevia and delicious fruits.

GIVE YOUR BODY A BREAK!

SEVEN FOODS THAT MAY OFFEND YOUR BODY

1. ANIMAL PROTEIN MAY OFFEND YOUR BODY

How does your body spend its time and energy? An important thing to realize about your body is that while it <u>creates</u> energy for you to function, it also <u>requires</u> energy to run well. **Animal Protein takes a lot of time and body energy to digest.**

50

Just like your car, your body needs the right kind fuel to operate efficiently. In her book, The Healing Power of Enzymes, Dr. DicQie Fuller, D.Sc. explains how a healthy person whose digestive system is working well requires about 80% of the body's energy simply for digestion. In other words, a healthy person who eats a healthy diet, digesting food takes more of your body energy than all of the other functions combined such as thinking, keeping your heart beating, breathing, creating hormones, cleansing and healing. The less healthy your diet, the more of your body energy goes to digestion and less to vital functions. It's no wonder so many Americans are tired all the time and can't seem to think clearly. All the energy needed for those functions is being used to digest the fast food they consume.

According to Lisa Cicciarello Andrews, College of Nursing, University of Cincinnati, red meats on average take from 1 to 3 days to be completely digested and eliminated from the body. Red meats take much longer to digest than other foods because of their high protein and fat content. (http://weight-loss-center.net/weight-loss-blog/2008/09/truth-about-red-meat-digestion/).

If your digestion is impaired by a weakened pancreas that does not excrete the proper amount of digestive enzymes,

the transit time for all cooked and processed foods, including meat will be longer.

Typical time from eating a meal to eliminating the waste from that meal is 16-24 hours, over 30 hours is not healthy. A folk medicine way to tell how quickly you are digesting your food is to eat several raw beets all at once. Write down the time you eat the beets and then check your next bowel movement. Continue to check your bowel movements until you see the red beet coloration, you will know how long it took to digest that food by the amount of time passed between eating them and when you notice them in your stool.

Our bodies receive nutrients from meat, but we also lose valuable energy for body function when we eat meats. In his book, Thrive, Brendan Frazier refers to this loss as negative energy nutrition. Conversely, raw vegetable and fruit juices take the least amount of time to digest; they are living foods and actually digest themselves with food enzymes contained in the food itself.

A raw apple contains living food enzymes that digest the apple in your stomach. You can see that when an apple on your counter becomes bruised, it begins to decay or "digest" itself, right there on your counter. A cooked apple, however, is dead food. The living enzymes are destroyed by heat so your body has to supply digestive enzymes from the pancreas to digest the cooked apple. Raw juices are easiest to digest because the fiber is removed. Transit time (from consumption to complete digestion) for freshly prepared living juice is 15 to 30 minutes. These take little energy away from the body so they are referred to as positive energy nutrition.

Protein from animal sources takes the most time and energy to digest. You can feel this when you eat large portions of meat at a meal, your energy lags for several hours as your

body puts its attention to breaking the meat and fat in the meat down so it can go through the small intestine where most nutrients are absorbed before being eliminated through the colon. Animal protein is a negative energy food and should be consumed in small quantities of excellent quality.

The animal protein you eat should come from animals that were fed good nutrition and are healthy. Conventionally grown beef, chicken, turkey, pork, fish and shellfish are not the meats your grandparents ate. They have poor nutrition themselves, are kept alive with antibiotics, and made to grow bigger and faster with hormones. Food Inc, The Movie, is a great source of information on what you are putting in your body. Does it make sense for you to eat food made from animals that are sick? Go to www.localharvest.org to find farmers in your area who grow healthy animals for meat. Health food market meats are a better choice if you must buy meat at the grocery store.

How much animal protein should you eat? A little is good for most people, Dr. Joel Fuhrman, MD, in his book Eat To Live, recommends reducing the amount of animal protein you eat to less than 12 ounces per week, yes per week. I know, you probably eat 12 ounce per day, most people do. 2 eggs for breakfast, 4-6 ounces of chicken for lunch and 4-8 ounces of red meat for dinner, potentially 10-16 ounces per day! Not to mention other animal proteins such as milk, yogurt, cheese, cottage cheese, ice cream most Americans consume on a daily basis.

Why does Dr. Fuhrman recommend such a small amount of animal protein? Dr. Fuhrman and other doctors and scientists who have studied health and nutrition have found that consuming too many animal products is the primary cause of heart disease, cancer and even type 2 Diabetes, the top three diseases in America today

T. Colin Campbell, Ph.D., in his book The China Study, conducted 40 years of research around the world studying indigenous people and their diet. He too found that cultures consuming a high amount of plant protein and little to no protein from animals did not suffer from the diseases we have in America.

Hallelujah Acres, a biblically based organization, has countless testimonials of people who have completely healed from cancer, diabetes, heart disease, depression, and many other chronic diseases as they eliminate all animal-based products from their diet.

Do you have to become a vegetarian for life? No, we don't recommend that to anyone. Eliminating or restricting the consumption of animal protein during your detox allows your body to put full effort towards cleansing and healing and less towards digestion. You will experience more energy and when your detox is complete you can decide how much animal protein you really need.

The FDA has not established guidelines for recommended daily allowances of protein. The Atkins Diet craze conditioned Americans to accept the over consumption of animal proteins. In the past people may have eaten animal protein every day but in much smaller quantities. I am in my fifties at this writing. I recall a large family eating a whole chicken for dinner and having left over's. Today, a couple may consume an entire rotisserie chicken at one sitting. Restaurant portions have also contributed to our over consumption of everything, including animal proteins.

How much protein do you need? Most health and nutrition professionals agree that humans need between 20 and 40 grams of protein per day. 1 cup of beans and 1 ounce of nuts and seeds is approximately 21 grams of protein and since everything, even lettuce contains some protein, there is really no problem getting enough protein from plants.

While you are detoxing be sure and eat plenty of plant protein from beans, nuts and seeds and reduce or eliminate animal protein.

When you reintroduce foods, consider keeping your animal protein to less than 12 ounces per week.

For more information on why animal protein is an offending food, read Eat to Live by Joel Fuhrman, MD and The China Study by T. Colin Campbell, Ph.D.

Ok, so you love your glass of wine or a beer every night (or is it 2 or 3 glasses), you need it to relax? Then you need coffee to get yourself up in the morning! People get most upset when starting the detox about giving up alcohol and caffeine! I think they may rather give up their first-born. I'm sure you have read magazine articles and heard news reports proclaiming the antioxidant benefits of red wine, coffee and chocolate, you know the polyphenols? Doesn't that make it good for you? Everything in moderation for a healthy body, however, if your body is not at prime function even good things can cause you problems. You can do anything for 28-days, even eliminating alcohol. Maybe you know in your heart that you are drinking just a little too much! (Or a lot). The next 28-days will bring some great revelation about your connection to many foods you now enjoy and alcohol is one of them.

Many times clients will say, "I had no idea how often I reach for a drink until I stopped drinking! I have so many connections to stress, loneliness, fatigue, social settings and alcohol I am amazed!"

There are some detox programs that allow you to drink alcohol moderately during the detox. Hmmmm.....mostly they do this because they think YOU don't have the will-power (or won't-power) to stop drinking for 28-days. Baloney! You can do ANYTHING for 28-days, right?

Remember what you are trying to accomplish during your detox. You are going to *Give Your Body a Break* from:

***Give Your Body A Break* from toxic foods:** Alcohol is extremely hard on your liver. Your liver is your primary detoxification organ. How much sense does it make to try to eliminate toxins and at the same time weaken your liver? That is like adding water to your gas because to save money. In a very short time you won't have to worry about how expensive gas is because you will be replacing your motor!

Give Your Body A Break **from digestion:** Alcohol is high in sugar; your pancreas really has to work hard to process it. It is cooked so it uses up lots of your precious digestive enzymes.

Give Your Body A Break **from toxic lifestyle habits:** Alcohol, like all other "addictives," can creep up, grab you from behind and hold on with a death grip! Taking a break for 28-days gives you new awareness about your connection to alcohol and gives you the opportunity to regain control!

Aren't these some great reasons to eliminate alcohol for a measly 28-day detox?

One more tidbit....there is a VERY STRONG connection to alcoholic tendencies and gluten sensitivity. Giving your body a break from both will provide some very interesting insight into what your body can handle!

What to drink instead of alcohol. You really won't miss the alcohol after about the first 3-5 days; however, if after 3-5 days you find you are still missing it, please search out help from Alcoholics Anonymous or Celebrate Recovery. Often people find themselves at a loss if you are at a cocktail party, dinner or other event where alcohol is a key component.

IDEAS TO HELP YOU AVOID ALCOHOL FOR 28-DAYS

1. **Avoid situations where alcohol will be served.** If you feel like it will be a problem for you to stop drinking, avoid places where you will be tempted, it's only 28-days!

2. **Drink something else.** You really don't HAVE to drink a beer or a glass of wine; this is a good time to overcome peer pressure. Choose mineral water and a lime or have the bartender make you a citrus beverage with mineral water but NO Grenadine! Ask for what you want! Tell the bartender you are on a detox and not drinking alcohol or sugar, see if they have ideas. Carry your Stevia with you, put in a few drops, stir with your straw or drink stirrer and suddenly you look just like everyone else.

3. **If you are at a social gathering where people are bringing food, bring your own mineral water.** We recommend Gerolstiener Mineral Water or Kombucha. It is naturally carbonated from the ground so you don't have the CO_2, which is bad for your health!

Just remember, sparkling mineral water with CO_2 (like Pierre) is acid forming, so it is only for a treat, not a regular event!

A great cookbook with non-alcoholic drink ideas is Sober Celebrations: Lively Entertaining Without the Spirits by Liz Scott. You can purchase it at www.amazon.com.

4. **If you end up realizing (or already know) that alcohol has too strong a grip on you**, there are some great groups to help. Most Cities have some AMAZING recovery programs that meet all over town day and night. They are attended by normal people who don't want alcohol to control their lives. Why not swallow your pride, overcome your fear and check it out? Most people who attend recovery groups enjoy them better than church. They are a safe and honest gathering of fellow strugglers. Do you really want to allow pride and fear

to rob you of the life you deserve? You will find information about gatherings in your area at these links:

Alcoholic's Anonymous www.alcoholicsanonymous.com

Celebrate Recovery www.celebraterecovery.com

3. CAFFEINE MAY OFFEND YOUR BODY

'We just value our morning coffee time together, I really don't see how we can give it up". Translation: "We love to take our addictive legal stimulants together in the morning; I don't see how we can give it up". Phil and I have found that we can enjoy talking and watching the sunrise with freshly made carrot juice, just like we did with coffee.

Caffeine from Coffee and Sodas is among the "acid forming foods". Acid forming foods cause inflammation, a major cause of degenerative disease. Your detox program is designed to alkalize your body and reduce harmful inflammation.

Caffeine can contribute to adrenal stress; essentially your adrenal glands are so overwhelmed by stress and caffeine that they are "blown out". A good way to tell if your adrenals are working correctly is when you have a "stress event". Your adrenals SHOULD respond by flooding your body with adrenaline to give you "super-human" power to deal with the stress event. If your adrenal glands are not working correctly or you have adrenal stress you will feel like you can't function at all; instead of being "super-human" you will feel like a wet dishrag.

Caffeine also causes insulin levels to rise, which in turn may hinder your ability to lose weight.

Remember What You Are Trying To Accomplish During Your Detox,:

Give Your Body A Break **From Toxic Foods:** Caffeine is extremely acid forming. The goal of the detox is to bring your body to an alkaline state, clear the body of toxins and stimulate your own body's detoxification system. Drinking coffee, decaf or soda will hinder this process.

You are also giving your adrenal glands a break from over-stimulation due to too much caffeine. A reasonable amount of caffeine on a non-detox diet would be 1(6 or 8 oz) cup per day, which is 60-100 mg of caffeine. If you get one tall coffee at Starbucks you have already exceeded that amount.

Many Natural Health experts agree you may experience the following symptoms if your adrenal glands are not working correctly.

These may be caused by poorly functioning adrenal glands
Fatigue
Decreased tolerance to cold
Poor circulation
Low blood sugar level (hypoglycemia)
Low blood pressure
Allergies
Apathy/lethargy
Depression
Low stamina
Low self-esteem due to low energy output
Aches and pains in joints
Low levels of gastric hydrochloric acid (which digests food in the lower portion of your stomach)
Tendency to constipation
Muscle weakness
Need for excessive amounts of sleep
Fear due to low energy and secondary copper toxicity

Lower resistance to infection
Subnormal body temperature

<< Replace caffeine with herbal teas or Teccino, a grain based caffeine free coffee. >>
Give Your Body A Break From Toxic Lifestyle Habits. Too much caffeine gives you the feeling you can do more than your body can actually handle. For many people, navigating an all too busy life is impossible without the use of caffeine. So let's be honest, what is the difference between that and being an alcoholic, speed or meth addict? Not much.

When you give up coffee for 28-days your body begins to return to normal function. The food you are eating nourishes all your organs and glands. You will begin to feel more energy than you had with all the coffee and soda and at night you will be TIRED and SLEEP! Yeah!

After your 28-days you will be able to decide if you want to add coffee back in and how much is truly reasonable.

4. CHEMICALS CONTAINED IN PROCESSED FOOD AND FOOD STORAGE CONTAINERS MAY OFFEND YOUR BODY

According to WHO (World Health Organization) many harmful chemicals show up in Human Mother's Milk. This is a little scary to me.

MSG is an extremely harmful food additive that is found in almost every processed food available. Many food cravings are due to MSG in the food. MSG is also very toxic to your body. It is in a category known as an "excitotoxin" which means it essentially causes brain cells to become so overactive they die. If you feel tired after eating out or eating packaged or processed foods, it may be you are getting MSG in your food. Brain fog anyone?

60

MSG is also known to increase high blood pressure, obesity, and diabetes and increases the appetite by up to 40%. MSG also counteracts the most often prescribed medications for high blood pressure called "Calcium Channel Blocker" because MSG acts as a calcium channel OPENER. It also can exacerbate autism and creates a valium-like GABA effect in otherwise healthy people.

Olestra (Olean)(the fat the body doesn't recognize as fat) this "fat free" additive attaches to vital nutrients and flushes them out of the body. OK...common sense people. This non-fat has a health hazard warning on the package, ever see it? This Product Contains Olestra. Olestra may cause abdominal cramping and loose stools. Olestra inhibits the absorption of some vitamins and other nutrients. Vitamins A, D, E, and K have been added. Need I say more?

BPA in plastics: "A study published in the September 17, 2008 edition of the Journal of the American Medical Association found that people with high concentrations of BPA in their urine had a higher risk of cardiovascular disease, type 2 diabetes and liver-enzyme abnormalities." To learn more about plastics in the kitchen check out http://www.seventhgeneration.com/learn/news/leachin-teach-guide-safe-plastics-kitchen this link provides lists of food storage containers that do not have BPA. Ziploc Baggies, Saran Wrap, Brita Pitchers and Pyrex are listed as safe.

5. DAIRY PRODUCTS MAY OFFEND YOUR BODY

What exactly is DAIRY? Anything from a cow! Ok, don't hit me! Why are dairy products an offending food?

After 2 years old the human body does not produce enough of the enzyme lactase, the milk enzyme, to process milk products. Many seasonal and food related allergies, colds and ear infections can be eliminated without medication, just by eliminating dairy products.

Modern, American commercial milk is genetically modified with known cancer causing hormones. Milk purchased from China contains melamine, which is known to cause kidney stones.

The PCRM (Physicians Committee for Responsible Medicine) released a statement that Milk is <u>not</u> good for you, in fact, poses more risks than benefits and initiated an investigation into the "milk mustache" ads. Citing According to the FDA:

"[C]ertain information is needed in the health claim in order for it to be truthful and not misleading to segments of the population that are not at high risk of developing osteoporosis or for whom no link between calcium and osteoporosis has been established."

Don't you need milk for strong bones? Check out another PCRM site http://www.strongbones.org .

If you are concerned about your family eating pasteurized dairy products (and you should be):

Reduce cow's milk consumption. Try Goat's Milk and Goat products like yogurt and cheese. Goat's milk is the closest in molecular structure to human milk and is more easily digested.

Read the labels and look for milk that is rBGH hormone free.

Organic Milk is a better choice if you are going to give milk to your family.

Look for milk that is non-homogenized. Homogenization means the fat is broken up into tiny particles. The particles are so tiny the body can't recognize them as fat and they are not digested. This can cause more health problems as undigested proteins and fats enter the blood stream.

In Their Own Words:

I can breathe! No more year round seasonal allergies! I can sleep! No more allergy or sleep medications! I never thought this would be possible but after eliminating dairy products for 21 days my allergies are completely gone, not even a little stuffy nose. I'll not be eating them again. The amazing thing is I did this for my wife; I thought she was the one who needed it. I've also lost 28 pounds male, 36

6. GRAINS AND ESPECIALLY WHEAT MAY OFFEND YOUR BODY

This was a big eye-opener for me. For many years I had suffered with eczema on my hands. My hands were so broken out and broken open that many times I would leave a trail of blood on papers or other items I picked up. My hands completely cleared up in the first week of my detox. It was amazing. Then, the first time I ate some bread, post detox, my hands broke out again, within about 10 minutes they started itching and by morning they were a mess. This was a very sad realization because I LOVE bread and products made with bread; however, I love not having pain all the time too, so pain-free won.

I completely eliminated all forms of wheat for about one year once I made this discovery. I was able to add spelt back into my diet in limited amounts. Finally, after four years, my hands no longer break out at all, even if I eat wheat. I still rarely eat it because something tells me it is just not for me. Today my hands are completely clear and look beautiful and young.

What is Gluten Intolerance and Celiac Disease?
You may be aware of the term "Gluten Intolerance", it has become somewhat of a fad, and however, it is a growing and serious health problem.   Gluten is a protein occurring primarily in four grains: Wheat, rye, barley and oats and is

present in all types of wheat such as whole grain wheat, wheat bran, spelt, triticale. Gluten is also present in all baked foods that are made from these grains: bread, pies, cake, breakfast cereals, porridge, cookies, pizza and pasta, thousands of processed foods contain Gluten, especially ones that are labeled "high protein". Many vegetarian protein replacement products are made from Sietan, which is wheat gluten.

Many people are intolerant to Wheat, Corn and Soy because of genetic modification and the starch content of modern grains. Modern wheat is 92% Starch and 8% protein. God made wheat to be 50% starch and 50% protein. Man made the change for greed sake and man suffers physically. We use Spelt, an ancient form of wheat because it maintains the original, God made starch to protein ration. Spelt is lower in gluten and contains an enzyme that helps to break down gluten; however, some people may not be able to tolerate spelt.

You will eliminate grains during the 21-day portion of your detox. You may have 1/2 cup of Quinoa each day during this time if you wish. Limit quinoa if you are concerned about weight loss. Clients who detox find long-term physical problems disappear when they eliminate wheat and gluten from their daily food.

In Their Own Words

I struggled with serious depression for many years. When I eliminated gluten from my diet my depression lifted, I am thankful for an answer! HH, 30+ female

"As soon as I added wheat back to my diet I began to itch all over my body. I thought, could that really be true? I tried it several times, and now know I definitely cannot handle wheat.

Now I understand some of the skin and colon problems I had for years, as long as I stay off all forms of wheat, including spelt, I am fine." NP, 51,F

My psoriasis completely goes away when I stay off all wheat and gluten. When I get busy and am not intentional about my food, my psoriasis returns and I am quickly reminded about what my body needs." LC, 55,F

Wheat not only offended my body, it offended my wife! She was happy when I added wheat back to my diet....one meal and we discovered wheat was the cause of my excessive gas! No more wheat for me!" JL, 36, M

7. REFINED SUGARS MAY OFFEND YOUR BODY

This is another hard one for many people to let go of. The average American eats approximately 148 pounds of sugar each year. Think about it, that is over half a cup per day! Refined sugar causes inflammation and inflammation sets your body up for disease. Many muscle type injuries could be healed quickly if the person went completely off all refined sugar products. The inflammation is eliminated and the tissue can heal.

During your detox you are to completely avoid all refined sugars and only eat natural sugars. Words for sugar include: cane syrup, dehydrated cane juice, organic cane juice, and words ending in dextrin and dextrose to name a few.

Where do you get your sugar? Most of your sugar intake comes from High Fructose Corn Syrup! "They", the greed-driven food companies are using American's willingness to believe what they see on TV to lie to us once again. Commercials "talking about" high fructose corn syrup are telling Americans, "There's nothing wrong with it, its corn!" Give me a break, ARE YOU KIDDING ME???

Of COURSE High Fructose CORN Syrup is Corn that has been genetically modified with the weed killer Round Up for starters. Corn that has been changed so much through years of modification that it is mostly starch and little in the way of nutrition. This mutated non-food is in pretty much all restaurant food and most prepared foods in the grocery.

What's wrong with High Fructose Corn Syrup? Well for starters just consider that it has been genetically modified with the DNA of Round Up. That means "they" take the DNA of Round Up and put it in the DNA of the corn seed. Have you ever sprayed Round Up on a weed? It is dead THE NEXT DAY! Round Up causes the cells of the weed, plant, or whatever it is sprayed on to literally explode. Your children are eating these dangerous chemicals in their ketchup, cold cereal, cookies, candy, soda pop, ice cream, and yogurt and juice, need I say more? Is it really worth it to give your kids that garbage or to eat it yourself?

High Fructose Corn Syrup is hard on your nervous system! From the book **"Are Your Kids Running On Empty?"** Ellen Briggs, Food Consultant & Sally Byrd ND, discuss "Corn" as an allergen among children:

*"The origin of corn syrup is corn. They are heavily processed to the point of removing any potential nutrients found in this plant. High-fructose corn syrup is created by applying high heat during the processing phase, which produces a free radical-filled end product. Consumption can cause notable stress on your children's bodily systems. By adding so much high-fructose corn syrup, corn syrup and corn sugar derivative sweeteners to so many foods and drinks, food manufacturers have added another negative consequence to food consumption, food allergies. **Research has determined corn to be a common allergy food among children. It is known to raise havoc in the circulatory and nervous systems of the young.** High-fructose corn syrup has proven to be a cheaper source of sweetener than refined sugar. Dr. Michael*

Gazsi points out, it is estimated that high-fructose corn syrup accounts for about 52 pounds per person per year of sugar consumption."

High fructose corn syrup has also been shown to be connected to a new condition showing up on many people's yearly physicals called, "elevated liver enzymes" which is a precursor to an all too common condition known as "Nonalcoholic Fatty Liver Disease", a precursor to the alcoholic version, cirrhosis of the liver. Imagine, you avoid alcohol due to its unhealthy effects your entire life and then are diagnosed with virtually the same liver disease as an alcoholic!

The Mayo Clinic website defines Non-alcoholic Fatty Liver Disease

"Nonalcoholic fatty liver disease is a term used to describe the accumulation of fat in the liver of people who drink little or no alcohol.

Nonalcoholic fatty liver disease is common and, for most people, causes no signs and symptoms and no complications. But in some people with nonalcoholic fatty liver disease, the fat that accumulates can cause inflammation and scarring in the liver. This more serious form of nonalcoholic fatty liver disease is sometimes called nonalcoholic steatohepatitis. At its most severe, nonalcoholic fatty liver disease can progress to liver failure"

An article in Business Week magazine cites a study done at Duke University connecting Non-alcoholic Fatty Liver Disease and the consumption of High Fructose Corn Syrup.

"We have identified an environmental risk factor that may contribute to the metabolic syndrome of insulin resistance and the complications of the metabolic syndrome, including liver injury," Dr. Manal Abdelmalek, associate professor of medicine

in the division of gastroenterology/hepatology at Duke University Medical Center and leader of a team of scientists behind the new research, said in a university news release.

The researchers examined the medical records of 427 adults with non-alcoholic fatty liver disease (NAFLD), along with questionnaires the patients completed about their diets.

Only 19 percent of adults with non-alcoholic fatty liver disease said they never drank beverages containing the sweetener; 29 percent did so every day, the investigators found.

"Non-alcoholic fatty liver disease is present in 30 percent of adults in the United States," Abdelmalek said in the news release. "Although only a minority of patient's progress to cirrhosis, such patients are at increased risk for liver failure, liver cancer, and the need for liver transplant. Unfortunately, there is no therapy for non-alcoholic fatty liver disease. My hope is to see if we can find a factor, such as increased consumption of high-fructose corn syrup, which if modified, can decrease the risk of liver disease." Business Week, March 22, 2010, Duke University Medical Center, news release, March 18, 2010.

This article states *"unfortunately there is no therapy for non-alcoholic fatty liver disease"*. Dr. Sandra Cabot, M.D., author of Raw Juices Can Save Your Life and an expert in natural ways to accomplish liver cleansing disagrees. In an article, Dr. Cabot reassures there is hope for healing fatty liver disease. She states *"many have reversed fatty liver disease and it's precursor, elevated liver enzymes by going through a body detox program* (like our Give Your Body A Break detox), *consuming freshly made vegetable juice and eating a whole foods, non-processed diet."*

In Their Own Words

"It's definitely the refined sugar. During the detox my skin was perfectly clear, no acne or outbreaks of any kind. I treated myself with candy made with refined sugar and the next day my face was a mess, completely broken out. Now I know I don't need expensive creams or facial treatments; I need to avoid sugar...completely!" MM, 46 yr. old female

WHAT TO USE INSTEAD OF REFINED SUGAR
DURING DETOX

Stevia is an herb that does not cause your blood sugar to spike and actually heals your pancreas! Use Stevia in drinks, get the liquid kind, it lasts longer and tastes better.

Raw local honey and raw Agave Nectar Use it SPARINGLY in place of sugar in drinks and desserts. Your body cannot handle more than 1 teaspoon 2-3 times per day.

ONLY USE ORGANIC RAW AGAVE NECTAR as other non-raw agave nectar is just like high fructose corn syrup in your body.

SWEETENERS TO USE AFTER DETOX

Raw Honey can be used in baking, drinks and desserts. Raw honey from your local area (within 100 miles) can help you overcome seasonal allergies by boosting your immune system. If you have allergies in the spring use a local raw clover honey. If you have allergies in the fall use local wildflower honeys. You can find local raw honey at www.localharvest.org

Rapadura or Sucanat is the least refined forms of cane sugar USE IT SPARINGLY, less than one time per month! Can be used like regular sugar but will take a little longer to dissolve.

Stevia is always a good choice, only use pure Sweet Leaf Stevia, others have corn or cane sugar added to them.

In Their Own Words

Ten-year-old Micah and his mother Dawn were helping at a group presentation in Brentwood, Tennessee. Micah and his two sisters, ages four and fourteen and his parents, in their early forties, had been on our Give Your Family a Break Detox and changed to a healthy, mostly raw food diet in months prior. The family lost over 100 pounds in just over 2 months and mom reversed her Type 2 diabetes diagnosis.

Micah and his sisters and parents had lived on the SAD (Standard American Diet) their entire lives and struggled with weight issues even as children. Micah's favorite food was pop tarts.

Micah and his mom joined me at this teaching session to tell their story and help with the food preparation. Micah was thrilled to learn from Kay, a grandmother aged woman, how to quickly peel carrots for juicing and he was eager to teach the class how to do this. His participation and enthusiasm was catching.

I was speaking to the class and said "taste is acquired, not intrinsic; texture is the main issue when you change foods. If you keep eating the good foods you will acquire a taste for them" Micah was sitting behind me on the stage and piped up *"that is absolutely true, that is what happened to me!"* I asked him to come up and share his experience.

"When I first started eating carrots, I hated them. But I just kept eating some every day. Now I really like them! "

He then picked up a huge carrot and began munching it down. Thank you Micah for making the point so well!

CHAPTER 4 HOW TO START EATING PEOPLE FOOD

Hopefully by now you are convinced you need to do something different. Doing a body detoxification program, like our Give Your Body a Break Detox is like jumping in the deep end of the pool to learn to swim. Some people do well with that; others prefer to start slowly. If you are a "jump in the deep end" type then read through the detox program, set a start date, make sure you have your plan and jump! Everyone should do a body detoxification at some point.

If a slow start feels more comfortable for you then that is what you should do. You'll be very successful. Everyone must adapt to life change, whether they take one step at a time or jump in the deep end.

MAKE HEALTHY CHANGES ONE STEP AT A TIME

Start with one change, when you get that change under your belt, add another. Work on yourself first; you can't enforce changes in your family until you have experienced the benefits for yourself.

Your Family will eventually follow your example. Don't nag, threaten or even talk about changes with them in the beginning, wait for them to ask you. Don't spend every meal looking longingly at their junk or feeling sorry for yourself that you aren't eating it. This new "food life" is a gift; you may be saving your life and the lives of your loved ones.

Grasp it as a gift and just do it yourself. Your family and friends will ask questions, they will want to try your food and eventually you will be slightly miffed because they will eat all your good food and leave you with the junk! Treat this change as an adventure and they will want to join you.

<< *Don't Give Up: Experts agree, children may need to try a new food ten to fifteen times before it will be accepted. Sometimes this even applies to adults!* >>

When you make changes to family food, do it sloooowly. Our clients who have the best results converting the family do it slowly and intentionally. They replace one meal each week with one of our healthy recipes. They slowly replace treats, mix spelt and wheat flour, almond milk and cow's milk, just a little at a time until no one even noticed the complete change.

Those of you who have children may remember when your kids were babies and you started feeding them "real" food. You had to coax, talk about how yummy it was, eat it yourself, several and sometimes MANY times before the food would be accepted. Experts agree it takes 10-15 times for a child to accept a new food (this can be especially true for an older child like, let's say, a 40 year old spouse).

Keep at it, be determined, you would not intentionally let your child eat poison, right? Even if they wanted to and threw a screaming fit or refused to eat anything else, you would remain strong because you love and care about your child. You have the wisdom to make good food choices; your child does not have that ability, until you TEACH them how.

Kids are more willing to change than you might think!

When we work with families, its mom and dad that have more resistance to giving up their favorite foods than the kids. *Adults get their pleasure from food but kids get their pleasure from LIFE!* We should take a lesson!

10-year-old Jocelyn wanted to read our book with her mom. Sometime later, Jocelyn began coaching her best friend Mallory on a detox, they started by eliminating sugar! Now they want to learn to eat more healthy foods!

If you recall our story, when I was 13 my mother completely changed our family food, virtually without warning. She wasn't a drill sergeant; she just didn't have anything else available. I knew it was "healthy" food but I don't remember being told the reason behind the sudden changes.

My rebellious reaction, which by the way had nothing to do with my parents, rebellion was my choice, was to "eat whatever I wanted, when I wanted to eat it". However, true to the scripture, "train up a child in the way they should go and when they are old they will not depart from it", when I asked God for help with my health and my food, He sent it and it turns out, Mom was right again!

Your children will follow what you truly believe in your heart to be truth, sooner or later. We started our healthy way of life after our kids were grown and gone but now, as they have seen we really believe in this and truly practice it, both our daughter Jesi and our son Robb have adopted some of our healthy lifestyle principles for themselves and our grandsons.

Start eating more real food, take one of these steps at a time, then, when you feel confident and enthusiastic and begin the next step. This process is simple, set a goal of one to two weeks for each step.

*<< **ONE STEP AT A TIME:** 1. Drink Water 2.Eat raw fruit for breakfast 3. Get your bowels moving each morning 4. Add 1 raw veggie to lunch and dinner 5. Snack on fruit and nuts 6. Eat sprouted grains, nuts and seeds 7. Eat some beans every day >>*

1. Drink Filtered water. Drink a good spring filtered water, no vitamin filtered waters or sports drinks. If you don't like the taste of filtered water, try adding some fresh lemon or lime juice. A pitcher filter is also a good choice. The best filters are ionizing filters, see Chapter 19.

2. Only eat fresh, raw fruit in the morning until your first bowel movement. I suffered with constipation for years. I thought it was normal to only have a bowel movement every few days. The truth is you were created to have a bowel movement after every meal. Think of your baby or your dog, eat and poop, eat and poop, yes, that should be you too.

According to thousands of years of tradition in Chinese medicine and more proof in modern natural medicine, your body detoxifies each organ in approximately 3-hour cycles.

The colon finishes its cleansing cycle about 7 am and that cycle should end with a bowel movement.

Essentially, while you sleep your body is cleansing each organ and moving the debris, toxins, etc, to the colon to be removed, much like cleaning house and taking out the trash.

The end of the colon cycle is to eliminate the trash through a bowel movement. If you eat a big breakfast before this elimination happens, you are stopping the colon cleansing cycle until it begins the next morning about 4 am.

You may have experienced eating a big heavy breakfast early in the morning and feeling like it is sitting there all day, well it most likely is because that big breakfast stopped the cleansing cycle and started the digestion cycle.

3. Get your bowels moving each morning. People should have a bowel movement each morning shortly after rising from a good night's sleep. If you don't there is a simple folk remedy that works for many people... Only eat fresh fruit until you have a bowel movement, *even if it takes all day, just eat fresh fruit. Eat fruit and drink lots of water with lemon juice.* After your bowel movement then begin to eat other healthy foods such as vegetables, and lots of leafy greens. Also try a flax seed smoothie. Follow this pattern each day until your body resets, you should find a good change in no more than 2-3 days. *A probiotic supplement may also help this process.*

We like Udo's Choice Probiotics or Garden of Life Primal Defense Probiotic. Many people have reversed constipation using this method. You may feel light headed or headachy at first, especially if you are used to coffee in the morning. These are usually symptoms of detoxifying and withdrawals, it may help to drink lots of water, eat juicy raw fruits.

It Works!: "Constipated most of my life, I tried the fruit only until your first BM, now I am no longer constipated!" F, 50+

4. Eat Raw Fruits & Veggies. Add 1 raw fruit to breakfast and 1 raw veggie to each lunch and dinner. If you want to start right away because you are enthusiastic, go ahead and start incorporating more raw foods like salads into your daily food. Even just adding 1 raw thing to each meal is a great first step. There are some great recipes in this book; a favorite is the Aunt Celeste's Kale Salad in Chapter 12.

Snack on fresh fruit. When you need a snack, reach for your favorite raw fruit instead of candy or cookies.

5. Eat Sprouted Grains, Nuts and Seeds. Get sprouted grain bread like Ezekiel or Alvarado Street Bakery. You can find them in the freezer section of most grocery stores, Health food markets and on the web. Eat 1 ounce of raw soaked nuts each day. See How To Soak Nuts and Seeds in chapter 15.

6. Eat Beans every day. Start eating a cup of cooked beans each day, any way you like them. There are many recipes in this book or just throw some on a salad.

REPLACE HARMFUL FOODS WITH GOOD FOODS

WORK ON THESE NEXT

1. Replace caffeine loaded drinks and sodas with Green Tea or Herbal Tea and work towards eliminating caffeine in your diet. Do it slowly so you don't get sick. You may go through withdrawals so start at a time when you can afford to not feel so great. Cut back by half each day and you'll quickly wean yourself from caffeine.

2. Replace alcohol. Once the caffeine is gone, eliminate alcohol. Just like caffeine, cut back slowly. You can replace it with mineral water.

3. Replace all refined sugar products with fruit. For most of us conditioned to eat fast food or boxed food, this step is challenging.

As you start to look more closely at the ingredients of your food, located on the food label, you'll notice some form of refined sugar in almost every processed item on the market.

Read the labels closely and make a plan to eat half as much sugar today as yesterday.

<< *Go to the next level!:* Choose Caffeine Free. Reduce Alcohol. Eat natural sugars. Eat sprouted, whole grains. Eat mostly plant proteins. Eat mostly fresh, raw foods. >>

Begin this weaning process as you do the others, by first reducing and then replacing any processed sugar (glucose, fructose, syrups) with living fresh fruits. A good encouragement is to choose fruit you really enjoy; you will feel like the fruit is a treat! Finally, keep in mind that sugar also includes sugar substitutes such as Sweet & Low, Equal, Splenda and all their generic brands.

4. Replace your wheat-based breads, pastas, crackers and cereals. Switch your breads and cereals from wheat-based products to sprouted breads like Ezekiel bread or Alvarado Street Bakery bread, organic corn chips, rice and seed crackers. Access our blog through the website for a running pantry list of things we enjoy on a regular basis.

5. Replace meat, fish, eggs, poultry and seafood with beans at least 3-5 times a week. Begin to reduce your animal protein to less than 12 ounces per week. This means all red meat, fish, shellfish, turkey, chicken, pork, milk, cheese, yogurt, cottage cheese, kefir, and lunchmeats.

To lessen your risk of the top three killers in America, Heart Disease, Cancer and Type 2 Diabetes, Dr. Joel Fuhrman, Eat to Live, recommends reducing the consumption of foods that comes from an animal, to a total of less than 12 oz. per week.

The China Study, by T. Colin Campbell, Ph.D., a 40-year study of food and disease in China and the Philippines, revealed that cultures who had little to no animal protein as a regular part of their diet had little to no incidence of the American diseases of cancer, heart disease, and Type 2 Diabetes. The recipes and meal plans in this book will help you do that.

<< *Go to the next level!: Eat People Food!*

Start Slowly. Drink Water. Eat Real Food. Mostly Plants >>

6. Replace all prepared foods with real, fresh foods. Eliminate chemicals from your diet such as artificial sweeteners like Equal, Splenda, high fructose corn syrup, read the ingredients on your labels. Start reducing the amount of processed foods you eat. These contain many chemicals that are addictive and harmful to your body. You will find delicious "treat" recipes we enjoy in this book.

SWITCH TO PEOPLE FOOD

It's not hard, it's just different and it will require you to use your brain and think about what you are going to eat and where you are going to get it. If you are going to eat well and *Give Your Body a Break* and vastly improve your health, you have to have a plan and work the plan. It's not hard; it's just different.

PLAN TO CHANGE

Any change requires a plan of action. You are about to make changes that will impact every area of your life. Up until now you have been able to stop at any city corner and find something to put in your mouth, chew and swallow. The food manufacturers call it "food" but it is usually just a bunch of chemicals with the flavor of food. Beware! Chemicals can be toxic and dangerous when ingested.

This book is designed to help you follow a plan to better eating and better health until you develop your own plan for your life. We have shared our daily food menus and even ideas for company and family favorites.

ONE STEP AT A TIME WILL GET YOU TO YOUR GOAL OF A TRULY HEALTHY BODY!

- *Plan your menu for the week. If that seems like too much, start with planning for the next day. Once you get that down, go for three days and then the whole week.*

- *Make a weekly appointment with yourself for menu planning and keep it instead of a doctor's appointment! Be sure you include drinking filtered water in your daily plan.*

- *Make a shopping list from your menu plan.*

- *Shop for your food. Follow your list, don't wander; you will spend too much money and too much time.*

- *Bring your food home and wash it, do your prep and follow your daily eating plan!*

WASH YOUR VEGGIES

Do you **really** need to wash the vegetables and fruits you bring home from the store? Your veggies look pretty clean when they come home from the grocery store, right? What you may not see is the animal, insect or human excrement on your fruits and veggies. Of course, there are also the pesticides, fertilizers and wax to name a few of the harmful chemicals.

We do not buy an expensive veggie wash. The veggie wash recipes in this book are quick, easy and accomplish the same goal, clean fruits and veggies without the tremendous expense. Make up a bottle of Spray Veggie Wash for quick cleans, like an apple you just brought in and want to munch on while doing your prep. Use the Raw Apple Cider Vinegar Veggie Wash or the Hydrogen Peroxide Veggie Wash to wash all your veggies at once. You will be shocked at what is left in the sink from those veggies that look "clean"!

HOW TO QUICKLY AND EFFICIENTLY WASH YOUR VEGGIES

Fill your sink with cold water and the veggie wash of your choice. Put your veggies in the sink, all of them together and allow them to soak for 30 minutes. Do this as soon as you bring them home from the grocery or market. You can put carrots, apples, lemons, and kale all together. If you have produce in the little boxes with holes or in bags with holes, like raspberries, cherry tomatoes or grapes just put the box or bag and all in the sink, no need to remove them.

Remember the old dish drainer we used to put our dishes on after hand washing? Get it out and pile your clean veggies on it, allow them to air dry out before storing. Simple!

DO NOT PREWASH Onions, Potatoes, Sweet Potatoes or bananas and avocados.

½ cup Braggs Raw Apple Cider Vinegar (yes, it must be raw) and a sink full of cold filtered water.

HYDROGEN PEROXIDE VEGGIE WASH

Least Expensive. **Pour** ½ cup hydrogen peroxide in a sink full of cold filtered water. Put your veggies in and allow soaking for 30 minutes, rinsing well. Research published by the Journal of Food and Science in 2003 showed effective results when using hydrogen peroxide to decontaminate apples and melons that were infected with strains of E coli.

SPRAY VEGGIE WASH

Just add a 2-4 Tablespoons of Braggs Raw Apple Cider Vinegar to a bottle of clean filtered water. Shake well, spray on veggies and then wash under flowing clean water as usual. This method helps to clean those fruits and veggies better than ever, and it's a lot less expensive than those commercial produce washes. Especially use this for grapes! Keep a brush handy for the root veggies like carrots and potatoes and beets.

In Their Own Words

Three years ago I was 19 years old, 299 pound, suicidal and on the verge of being a diabetic and having high blood pressure. My weekly diet consisted of frozen chicken nuggets, canned green beans and corn, and boxed meals like Hamburger Helper. At least 2x a week I suffered with headaches, chest pains, and/or breathing difficulty.

During the detox, I changed my diet dramatically. The most significant change I made was switching from processed foods to raw foods. My diet went from being 5% raw foods to 75-90% raw foods.

Now I'm 24 years old, 180 pounds, and my blood pressure is normal. I have no more chest pains, or breathing difficulty, and the headaches only come when I eat processed foods that aren't good for me. My weekly diet now consists of a variety of salads, including spring mix, veggie romaine, or (my new favorite) spinach and quinoa salad. I also eat a variety of fruits and nuts...I even make my own healthy, unprocessed, and unbreaded chicken strips. EP, F, 22

CHAPTER 5   SETTING UP YOUR KITCHEN

If you are going to eat real food you are going to have to prepare it but don't worry, helping with your preparation is what this book is all about! The equipment we suggest can make your prep time a whiz. You may already have some of these tools on hand. If you don't have the particular brand we recommend, use what you have until you are able to replace it with a better option.

Many people start by asking friends and family members if they have some of this equipment around they aren't currently using. This works well until your friends and family see how great you look and feel, then they want theirs back. My sister-in-law was using her mother's champion juicer, which she had not used in about 10 years. She kept sharing her great progress with her mother and soon she was informed she needed to get a juicer of her own. She was happy her mom was getting back to health so my sister-in-law found a used one for a great price on Craig's list.

Juicers should be the first replaceable item as mainstream juicers often "expire" from regular use. The type of juicer you use determines the nutritional value of the juice you get from your fruits and vegetables; this is very important.

√ **A Juicer:** You must have a good one. We recommend the Champion or the Green Star.

√ **Food Processor:** Our Favorite is the Kitchen Aid 12 cup food processor.

√ **A magic bullet**, high-speed blender or immersion blender stick.

√ **A vegetable peeler** and at least one good, sharp knife you can sharpen frequently and a cutting board.

√ **Glass storage containers.** These can be accumulated as you go. Start with what you have, even if it's plastic, but work towards replacing plastic containers with glass.

√ **A pantry stocked with staples.** We have included a tear out "Pantry List" at the back of this book.

√ **A freshly stocked spice cabinet** with a few of your favorite spices.

√ **Basic kitchen equipment** like good knives, measuring cups and spoons, scrapers and tongs.

√ **A convection oven** that will replace your microwave, read on to learn more about the dangers of microwave ovens.

EXTRAS THAT ARE NICE BUT NOT IMPERATIVE

Dehydrator, although I prayed for one and believe God brought it to me, I rarely use it as I don't have the time or desire (PS: I don't want to sell it. Sorry).

A Blendtec or Vita Mix high-speed blender.

Kitchen Aide Mixer in case you decide to make your own bread, this makes it easier, although I have made bread weekly using a large glass bowl and a heavy spoon.

A grain mill in case you want to grind your own flour (Grinding flour may not be the first food preparation process you want to try right away).

What if you don't have the money to buy any or all of this equipment?

Ask God to give you what you need. This is how I got my dehydrator, my first food processor and my juicer! One client was GIVEN a Champion Juicer by her bug exterminator.

Email your friends, post an inquiry on Face book such as "I need a food processor" and chances are you will receive offers from folks wanting to clean out their closet or garages.

Other good resources are the local Good Will stores, garage sales, Craig's List and EBay. It's not unusual for us to have people in our Whole Foods cooking classes using their "i-phones" to bid on juicers during class.

SET UP YOUR KITCHEN

Our philosophy is kitchens are for cooking, not for looking cool. Seriously, making your food is not going to be fun if you don't have the adequate room. Clear off all the counters. Put the papers where papers belong, put the knick-knacks somewhere else, you are going to USE your kitchen.

WHAT SHOULD BE ON YOUR KITCHEN COUNTER?

Your food processor.

Your juicer.

Your convection oven (unless you have one built in).

85

Any equipment you use daily like your blender or magic bullet.

A counter top container for frequently used tools like scrapers and spatulas.

Lots of empty counter space for food prep.

A basket for fresh fruits and veggies.

If you really want to do it right, take everything out of your kitchen cabinets and give away the equipment and utensils you don't use. One client, who did a "kitchen makeover", had a whole room of pans, dishes, gadgets to give away and a box full of fancy cooking tools that had never been opened. Another client was ecstatic to find a whole new counter for food preparation when she created an organized space to keep important papers and miscellaneous items in her pantry.

Sink area: This area is for food prep and cleanup. A drainer to put your veggies on after you wash them, a spot for your veggie wash, brushes, peelers, colanders.

Stove area: This area is for cooking; put your cooking tools here and staples, including spices, oils, packages of beans, pasta, and canned food that gets heated, etc. You can put cans and packages of food in your pantry but keep your spices and oils in a cabinet near the stove but away from heat.

Food Prep area: This area is for your juicer, food processor, magic bullet, mixer, knives and cutting boards. You will also want any gadgets you use, like a garlic press, mandolin, hand grater, and citrus juicer in this area. Put your food storage containers, zip loc bags and Baggies, juice jars, mixing bowls, measuring spoons, wire whisks in cabinets or drawers close by.

WHY MAKE YOUR OWN JUICE?

The point of juicing is to get living enzymes, which facilitate repair into the cell as quickly as possible. Removing the pulp (fiber) from the juice allows the nutrients to be absorbed into the blood stream from the small intestine as opposed to being absorbed through the colon. Freshly extracted vegetable juice is digested quickly in the stomach and moved into the small intestine in about 20 minutes, as opposed to 2-6 hours to go through the entire digestive process.

According to Steve Mack, Children's Hospital Oakland Research Institute, approximately three million of your cells die each second. As a cell dies, it creates an exact replica of itself. When you juice, the cells are flooded with the enzymes, phytonutrients, minerals and vitamins of the veggies or fruits you juice. As those enzymes and nutrients enter the dying cell, it is cleansed and fortified so the new cell it creates will be stronger than the original cell. If you continue to drink the freshly extracted vegetable and fruit juices your cells will continue to become stronger and healthier instead of weaker. Dr. H. Norman Walker, D.Sc, wrote a book "Becoming Younger" his story of healing and living to over 100 years of age. He attributes his long life and great health after the age of 50 years old to drinking large quantities of freshly extracted vegetable juices.

The enzymes are fragile in oxygen and heat. It is very important to use a juicer that protects the living enzymes in the food. RPM's, revolutions per minute, are responsible for damaging the living enzymes. It is important to get a juicer with low RPM's. Juicers should not be chosen for cost but for the quality of juice the extract.

Centrifugal juicers -5,000 – 10,000 RPM's

Any juicer is better than no juicer. You will find these in Department Stores and sold on TV.

Centrifugal juicers, have baskets that spin around little knives, cutting the food and producing juice. The juice is exposed to a great deal of heat as it whirs through the basket. Examples of Centrifugal juicers are Juice Man, Jack La Lane and Breville. These types of juicers yield the least amount of juice per pound. They are also the least expensive. Juice made from these juicers will have less living enzymes and must be consumed within 18 minutes of making the juice.

Masticating juicers -1,800 RPM's

We use a Champion and sell them, check out the store on our website for more information.

Masticating juicers have cone shaped knives that cut the vegetables and extract the juice. The juice goes quickly through the cutter and is not exposed too much heat, which destroys the enzymes. Examples of a masticating juicer are Champion and Omega juicers. We use a champion a daily basis. We get twice as much juice from our champion as others report from a centrifugal juicer. Juice made in a masticating juicer can be kept in a sealed glass jar, filled completely to the top of the jar, for up to 24 hours.

Extraction or Gear Driven juicers -110 RPM's

Best Choice Green Star, buy from us and we'll teach you how to use it too, www.thewellnessworkshop.org

Extraction juicers use gears to press the juice out of the food. They run at extremely low RPM's and are proven to extract a substantially higher quantity of minerals than the other types of juicers. Concentrations of essential minerals, like calcium, iron, and zinc are 50%-200% higher in juice from an extraction juicer. People with cancer or other diseases that are using freshly extracted juices to heal the body should only use an extraction juicer. Studies done by the Gerson Clinic, a world renowned natural health clinic who have helped thousands of people heal from all types of disease including cancer, show that patients using other types of juicers do not experience dramatic healing until they switch to an extraction juicer. A significantly higher yield, higher enzyme retention and the ability to keep the juice for up to 72 hours make this type of juicer a good choice. Green Star juicers are extraction juicers.

<< *Centrifugal Juicer:* Drink the juice immediately *Masticating Juicer:* Drink immediately or store in a sealed jar in the refrigerator for up to 24 hours *Extraction Juicer:* Drink immediately or store in a sealed jar in the refrigerator up to 72 hours. >>

STOP USING YOUR MICROWAVE

Micro-waved Food May Be Hazardous to Your Health

We do not use our microwave and have not used one at all for over three years. This is probably the hardest change we had to make, harder than giving up candy! Microwaves are convenient and we are always looking for convenience. I was able to break the habit by filling our built in microwave with things I never use, to make it too difficult to use it. Now we don't own a microwave, nor have a built in microwave in our kitchen. In addition to using a microwave in your home, all processed foods and most foods you buy in a restaurant are also prepared using a microwave oven.

Here are some reasons to throw out your microwave: Eating Micro waved food can cause permanent brain damage by shorting out electrical impulses in the brain, shut down male and female hormone production, prohibit your body from receiving the neurotransmitters that make you feel good, sleep well and have motivation. Microwaving affects the molecular structure of food, destroys up to 98% of nutrients in food and changes the fat in Micro waved meats into trans Fats. A full article about the dangers of micro waved food is found on Dr. Joseph Mercola's website, http://www.mercola.com/article/microwave/hazards.htm.

Use a Convection Oven Instead Of Your Microwave

Most people are used to the convenience of the microwave for reheating foods and drinks. We use a portable convection oven that sits on our counter for reheating foods, baking cookies and broiling. It only takes a minute or two longer and you completely avoid harmful radiation, the convection oven is also quicker and easier than using the stovetop and big oven.

Why Don't You Hear These Truths In The Media

If you are like me you had no idea about the food you eat. You thought if our government allows people to sell it to me to eat, it must be good for me. You thought the FDA was in existence to protect us from harmful food and drugs. We must face the truth. America is a capitalistic society, in other words, "it's all about the money". Corporate decisions about your health are likely based on someone making money, not necessarily on what is good for your body. Do you make decisions about your health based on money as well?

Let's look for just a minute at some of the industries supported by you and I consuming fast food.

- Packaging design and production
- Transportation (trucking)

90

- Construction of new buildings
- Design and construction of commercial food prep equipment
- Design and construction of packaging plants
- Design and construction of waste management facilities
- Mass farming
- Food science for preservation, preparation and flavor
- Industrial food preparation
- Automotive (drive through)
- Medical (from all the side effects of the bad food)
- Insurance (so you will go to the doctor)
- Construction of medical buildings
- Colleges and Universities that give us our doctors, dentists, food engineers, drug engineers, scientists, building and equipment engineers
- Advertising (which supports media)
- Television and movies (supported by advertising)
- Stock market (commodities like soy and corn)

Need I say more? Why would the very people who make money from you and I eating fast food want us to stop? Remember when Oprah Winfrey did a spot on the dangers of meat from feed yards back in the 1980's? The beef barons sued Oprah and her guest, Howard F. Lyman, author of <u>The Mad Cowboy</u>. Oprah won the lawsuit because everything she said was true; however, that suit spawned a federal law called the Food Disparagement law. It is against the law for anyone to speak against a food in a way that would prevent the food producer from making money. Crazy.

CHAPTER 6   CHOOSING PEOPLE FOOD

Reading the ingredients on food packages was a big change for us, but we learned it is one of the best things you can do for your health. Americans have been conditioned to read "Nutrition Facts" but not the ingredients. Honestly, it doesn't matter if your food is low sugar, low fat, low carb or high protein if it is poison to your body.

Our Rule: If it has more than 5 Ingredients we usually don't buy it. If it has more than 5, can you pronounce words? Are they real food that you would recognize like for instance, broccoli? A simple way to start is just to look for two ingredients: MSG and High Fructose Corn Syrup. If a food has either of those, just don't eat it and you will avoid most of the other harmful additives and preservatives.

WE READ THE LABEL INGREDIENTS AND AVOID THESE

Cow products have either or both Butylated Hydroxyanisole (BHA) and Butylated Hydroxytoluene (BHT)
Propyl Gallate
Sodium Nitrate/Nitrate (deli meats & processed meats/sausages)

Sulfites (Sulfur Dioxide, Sodium Sulfite, Sodium And Potassium Bisulfite, Sodium and Potassium Metabisulfite (dried fruit & raisins)

Potassium Bromate (white flour and white flour products)

FD&C Blue No. 1

FD&C Blue No. 2

FD&C Green No. 3

FD&C Red No. 3 (Erythrosine)

FD&C Yellow No. 5 (Tartrazine)

FD&C Yellow No. 6

Monosodium Glutamate (MSG)

Non-organic & Non-GMO Canola, Corn or Soy, Cotton seed oils and proteins

Sucrose................................. common table sugar
Glucose, Dextrose.......................corn sugar
Fructose................................. fruit sugar
Lactose................................. milk sugar
Maltose................................. malt sugar
Corn Syrup............................. sweetener made from corn starch
Honey................................. syrup of fructose and glucose
Molasses............................... concentrated sap of sugar bearing plants (sugar cane, sugar beets)
Brown Sugar..........................sucrose covered with small amounts of molasses
Maple Sugar.........................concentrated sap of sugar maple trees
Sugar Alcohols..........................sorbitol, mannitol, maltitol, and xylitol
High Fructose Corn Syrup (in everything from bread to pickle relish)
Chemical sugar substitutes: Acesulfame-K, Sucralose (aka: Splenda), Aspartame (aka: Equal, Nutra Sweet, Amino-Sweet))
All soda's with CO_2 which is known to cause bone loss and osteoporosis
All dried & liquid dairy substitutes such as dried and flavored coffee creamers
All forms of Peanuts and Peanut butter all of which have a cancer causing mold, which cannot be removed or controlled. (412 pesticide and chemical residues per serving). You may find interesting information in David Steinman's book Diet for a Poisoned Planet.

"Just because you can put it in your mouth, Doesn't mean its food!"

Cyndi Shalhoub, Organic Chef htpp://organicchefcyndi.com

CHOOSING "PEOPLE FOOD QUALITY"

MEAT, FISH AND EGGS

We discussed the importance of good quality animal protein in chapter two but it bears repeating; if you must choose between buying organic fruits and veggies and naturally grown or organic meat, poultry and fish, choose to buy natural animal products, your health depends on it.

You may be able to find special organically grown meats and eggs at the local grocery but be aware that their store brands are most likely going to be "factory-raised" so be sure to read the label. Whole Foods store brand is acceptable.

Why is quality meat so important? Beef, Chicken and Fish raised in commercial "factories" are subjected to growth hormones that are dangerous for your health and must receive antibiotics to prevent the diseases that flourish in those environments. Fish farms are so disease-ridden that 40% of the fish die before they can be harvested. What do they do with the diseased, dead fish? Grind them up and use them as feed and fertilizer for other forms of food. Really, how can that be right? Similar things happen in poultry, beef and pork "factories".

How to choose the right meat. Look for the terms "Organic, Hormone Free, Range Fed or Grass Fed" when it comes to Beef, Chicken, and Turkey. Always look for "Wild Caught" when it comes to Fish. The same is true for eggs. Organic, Hormone Free, Range Fed or Free Range eggs produce the best source of protein and Omega 3-6. Shrimp is predominately farmed, you will have to search for "wild caught" shrimp. The Tuna debate rages but if you are pregnant or have small children, you should definitely limit your tuna intake. Just one can per week can provide four times the allowable level of mercury ingested. Halibut is always wild caught and is a delicious option.

Shellfish, crustaceans and bottom fish (commonly called shrimp, crab and catfish) are the vacuum cleaners of the water. They are extremely toxic and should be avoided. Remember in the Old Testament God told His people not to eat these things. God was not trying to be mean; because He simply didn't create them for our food; their purpose is to clean the rivers, lakes and oceans. Eating those types of seafood is comparable to taking the filter out of your aquarium and serving it for dinner, deep-fried of course!

Processed meats: Lunchmeats, hot dogs, sausage, and ham are full of nitrites and nitrates that have many health consequences. You can find deli meat without additives and preservatives at your local health food market and some grocery stores. You can also find some sausage products, hot dogs and pepperoni that are nitrite free. Most major grocery chains are jumping on the "whole food" bandwagon and order from the same companies. They want your business and are willing to offer better choices at consumer request. If your local grocery store doesn't have what you are looking for, go to the Customer Service Desk and ask them to order it, you may need the specific name, brand and size you want to order.

POTENTIALLY DANGEROUS FOODS TO PEOPLE

Dried Fruits: On Detox use raisins and cranberries SPARINGLY (1 Tablespoon per day). Always read the label on dried fruits. Only buy organic dried fruits, even raisins. Dried fruits are sprayed with pesticides during processing, Good Grief! If it doesn't say "no sugar added & no sulphates or sulphites" then it most likely has all those things, don't buy it or use it. Dried fruits without sulphates and sulphites will not have a vibrant color but they are a better product. The brightly colored dried fruits are treated with these harmful chemicals.

Peanut Butter: This American staple is extremely toxic. The amount of toxins in the form of pesticides and chemical residues in our food and water is astounding. A great book for more information about foods that are less contaminated and foods you should absolutely avoid is **Diet for a Poisoned Planet**, by David Steinman.

One scary statistic reveals the contaminates in Peanut Butter. Besides containing a mold that is known to cause cancer, Aflatoxin, FDA tests revealed 413 contaminants in Peanut Butter, one of the highest toxicity levels of all foods and yet it is a staple for our children.

Use Raw Almond butter in place of peanut butter and buy a copy of **Diet for a Poisoned Planet** by David Steinman, to keep for a reference.

There are many good books and movies out as of this writing.

CHOOSING THE RIGHT OILS FOR PEOPLE

Only buy cold pressed or expeller pressed unrefined oils. This is especially important when purchasing coconut oil and olive oil. Olive oil and Canola oil convert to a trans Fat at about 250 degrees F so you should not cook or bake with them.

Coconut oil is a wonderful choice; it is antiviral and antibacterial and contains Lauric acid, which helps the body to process fat.

We avoid canola oil all together because it is one of the top four foods genetically modified with the weed killer, Round-up. It is also converts to trans Fat at a low temperature.

Flaxseed oil is the only oil that does not convert to body fat; we use it as much as possible in uncooked foods like salads and dressings. Do not cook with flax seed oil.

For more information on healthy oils and fats read <u>Fats That Heal, Fats That Kill</u> by Udo Erasamus.

WONDERFUL "NEW" PEOPLE FOODS

Continuing to eat well required us to expand our horizons or become VERY bored by eating the same things all the time. During our first 4 months, the time period when we lost a combined total of 132 pounds (oh sorry, did I say that already?), Saturday was our treat day. Each Saturday morning we enjoyed a cup of coffee together, usually on our deck. We also had a treat meal on Saturday, usually alternating between Pizza and Pancakes. I enjoyed something chocolate one time a month. The rest of the week we ate mostly salads, a lot of Phil's Famous Kitchen Sink Soup and stir-fry type dishes.

During that time we completely avoided anything with sugar, breads, pastas, cheese, and milk except for the Saturday treats. After about 6 months it became obvious that we needed some variety in our food so I began to search for natural foods to replace the ones we gave up. These are used in many of the recipes in this cookbook and are foods we enjoy on a regular basis.

Medjool Dates

Medjool dates are set apart from other drier forms of dates by their soft, chewy sweet texture. To store Medjool dates, leave them covered on the counter for up to a week or place them in an air-tight container in the refrigerator for up to six months. Pesticides are not generally used on Medjool dates. Eat them sparingly as treats; one date has 32 grams (equivalent of 8 teaspoons as sugar). While they metabolize differently than refined sugar and do not store as fat, too many dates eaten alone may cause you to have a drowsy glycemic reaction.

Why is it better? In addition to their high sugar content, Medjool dates add fiber, lots of potassium and B vitamins. Using them in baked breads and muffins produces a moist, chewy texture. Dates convert to sugar in the liver and do not store as fat! Dates are an alkaline fruit.

Where to get it? Many markets carry dates, however, the Medjool, which is the kind you should use in baking and raw treats, are a little more elusive. Warehouse stores usually carry them in the produce section as does your local health food market.

How do I use it? Use dates in place of brown sugar in baked goods such as muffins, cakes, cookies and bread. Blend pitted Medjool dates with a little water in your magic bullet to make a thick creamy paste and use about ¼ cup blended dates to 1-cup brown sugar. You may have to play with your recipe at first to get it right. Use dates in raw treats as the sugar. There are several recipes in this book that use Medjool dates.

As a work out energy boost, Medjool dates can't be beat. Keep one in your pocket to eat half way through your work out for quick recovery of energy, making them a much better choice than some type of refined sugar snack.

Coconut Sugar and Syrup

Coconut Sugar, our new favorite sweetener, is produced from the sweet juices of tropical coconut palm sugar blossoms. Raw coconut sugar is never heated above 90 degrees during processing so the enzymes are intact. Coconut sugar has long been a staple in South East Asian culinary heritage and herbal medicine.

Why is it better?
Coconut Sugar is rated as a GI 35. Honeys are GI 55 and Cane Sugars are GI 68. Coconut Sugar has a nutritional content far richer than all other commercially available sweeteners. Coconut Sugar is especially high in Potassium, Magnesium, Zinc and Iron and is a natural source of the vitamins B1, B2, B3, B6 and C. Coconut Sugar is a 100% Organic, unprocessed, unfiltered, and unbleached natural sweetener and contains no additives or preservatives.

Where to get it? Coconut sugar and syrup can be purchased on line and currently at Health food markets. The syrup is very sweet and sticky, it can be used in liquids or on pancakes, etc. The dried version is like a rich dark brown sugar.

How do I use it? Use coconut syrup like you would honey or agave nectar. It does not have a coconut taste at all. Use the crystals in place of any refined white or brown sugar.

Organic Raw Agave Nectar

Raw agave nectar, a natural sweetener, is extracted from a cactus like plant called the Agave Plant. It is mainly grown in Mexico and is an ingredient in Tequila. You can buy both raw and pasteurized versions.

Due to reports that sources of Raw Agave Nectar are compromised and some companies lace their agave nectar with corn syrup, we do not normally use this product. If you choose to use it be sure it is organic and raw.

Unrefined Cane Sugar Rapadura and Sucanat

There are two commercial brands of unrefined dehydrated cane juice; Rapadura and Sucanat. Of the two, I prefer Rapadura because it dissolves more easily in recipes.

Because these two sugars are unrefined, the appearance is like a small, coarse brown sand; quite different from white or brown sugar or even Dermera or Turbinado.

Sucanat and Rapadura are great sugar alternatives and offer the most nutritional value among all manufactured sweeteners. They're made from sugar cane juice that is clarified, filtered and evaporated. The remaining syrup is crystallized to create the wholesome sweeteners, which retain all the vitamins and minerals along with molasses and caramel flavor, making them excellent substitutes for any recipes that call for sugar.

Why is it better? Both Rapadura and Sucanat are generally accepted as a substitute for brown sugar. Unlike regular brown sugar, they are grainy instead of crystalline. Of all major sugars derived from sugar cane, Rapadura and Sucanat (not a "processed" sugar) ranks the highest in nutritional value, containing a smaller proportion of sucrose than white cane sugar. However, Sucanat (in common with all sugars) is not a significant source of any nutrient apart from simple carbohydrates.

Dr. David Reuben, author of Everything You Always Wanted to Know About Nutrition says,

"...white refined sugar-is not a food. It is a pure chemical extracted from plant sources, purer in fact than cocaine, which it resembles in many ways. Its true name is sucrose and its chemical formula is C12H22O11".

Where to get it? Most grocery stores carry either Rapadura or Sucanat in their health food area. Many times, if you ask at the Customer Service Counter, your grocery store will order anything you request. You can also purchase both Rapadura and Sucanat on line and at your local grocer and many health food stores.

How do I use it? Remember these are sugar and have very little nutritional value compared to fruits and vegetables. Use Rapadura and Sucanat for baked treats; less than one time per week. In baking, substitute equal amounts of Rapadura or Sucanat for brown sugar. Use raw, local honey or raw coconut sugar in place of white sugar.

You may need to run your mixer a little longer if you are trying to cream Rapadura or Sucanat as they do not dissolve as quickly as the white sugar you are used to. If you use these sugars in a product, you may notice a more brown or tan color due to the fact that they contain molasses.

Raw Local Honey

Honey is superior to sugar in that it has more vitamins and minerals, is sweeter, and raises one's blood sugar more slowly. It is unrefined and natural. It also will keep your baked goods moist longer.

Why is it better? Vitamins, nutrients and enzymes beneficial to the body are present and easily assimilated from raw honey. Processed honey (honey that has been heated over 119 degrees) has had these natural nutrients destroyed before the honey is packed in the jar.

Raw honey contains minerals, amino acids, enzymes, natural antioxidants, and vitamins. These healthy raw honey benefits can vary greatly depending on the flower source the nectar is gathered from. The study of spores and pollens in raw honey (known as melissopalynology) can determine the flower source of the nectar of every raw honey.

Raw Honey has health qualities that include antiseptic, digestion aid and promoting burn healing. Raw honey also contains many of the trace minerals needed to sustain a healthy body including selenium, phosphorous, zinc, chromium, potassium, iron, magnesium, copper, manganese and calcium.

Baking With Honey

NOTE TOTAL AMOUNT OF SUGAR IN RECIPE

TO REPLACE 1 CUP OF SUGAR:

¾ CUP PLUS 2 TABLESPOONS HONEY

ADD ¼ TEASPOON BAKING SODA

SUBTRACT 3 TABLESPOONS LIQUID (COULD BE MILK, 1 EGG, WATER, OR OIL)

REDUCE OVEN TEMPERATURE BY 25 DEGREES AND WATCH YOUR FIRST BATCH, AS HONEY WILL PRODUCE A BROWNER PRODUCT.

Where do I buy it? Your health food store, farmer's market and Health food market all should carry raw local honey. You can also go on line at www.localharvest.org. Locate the search box and enter raw honey; put your zip code in the appropriate box to view a list of local raw honey producers. Choose one that has several years experience.

How do I use it? Honey can be substituted for sugar in baked goods, puddings, pies and even drinks and salad dressings. Honey is sweeter than sugar so you can use less. Use honey in drinks, dressings, puddings, as you would sugar.

Stevia

Stevia is an herb and must be labeled as a supplement in the United States.

Why is it better? Stevia does not cause a rise in blood sugar and is a good choice for diabetics and those suffering with hypoglycemia. Stevia is known to heal the pancreas and reduce high blood pressure. It is 300 times sweeter than sugar and makes any sweetener it is combined with up to 100 times sweeter.

Where do I buy it? ONLY BUY PURE STEVIA. You will find it in the health food section of your health food store, not in the sweetener section. As health foods rise in popularity the mainstream food industry is combining Stevia with sugar, corn sugar, and non-sugar sweeteners as a marketing ploy. These forms of Stevia are not good for you. Pure Stevia can be purchased at most health food stores and in the health food section of most grocery stores, it is also available on-line. We prefer liquid Sweet Leaf Stevia; however it is available in packets.

How do I use it? You can use Stevia as you would sugar in any liquids. There are cookbooks specifically developed for

Stevia. It is important to use proper ratios and ingredients if you are going to bake with Stevia or use it in recipes. We do not have any recipes with Stevia in this cookbook.

To reduce sugar in a recipe: Stevia makes anything 100 times sweeter. Start a recipe with a little less sugar, honey or coconut sugar or agave nectar and add a little Stevia until it is the right sweetness for you.

HEALTHY OILS

All oils that are heated to excessive heats will become unstable.

Olive Oil

I absolutely love a fresh Olive oil, you won't find one in the grocery but there are sources in Chapter 19. Using the right oil the right way is vital to good health. The media and celebrity chefs promote the use of olive oil for cooking and many people now use olive oil, which is a heart healthy oil when used uncooked. Cooking olive oil above 250 degrees F makes the oil unstable, which is very damaging to the body.

The safe way to use Olive oil is uncooked, in salad dressings or added to pastas, sauces and soups just prior to serving.

Only purchase cold pressed or expeller pressed Olive oil. The more "virgin" the oil, the better the flavor, nutritional value and taste. Inexpensive Olive oil that is not cold pressed or expeller pressed is extracted using solvents and is not at all healthy. Read the label for the words "cold pressed" or "expeller pressed".

106

NOTE: Olive Oil is heart healthy oil as long as it is used without heating it.

Grape seed Oil

Grape seed oil, a vegetable oil, is a by-product of pressing grapes for wine.

Why is it better? Grape seed oil is known to lower cholesterol, can tolerate heat up to 485 degrees F without becoming unstable. Olive and Canola oil become unstable at about 250 degrees F. Grape seed's neutral flavor takes on the flavors of the food instead of your food tasting like oil. It mixes well and does not separate. This oil does not turn cloudy when refrigerated. We use Grape seed oil for almost everything.

Where do I buy it? Most grocery stores carry Grape seed oil in their health food area. You can also get it on line and at Health food markets and many health food stores.

How do I use it? Anytime you would use vegetable, canola or olive oil use Grape seed oil in equal amounts.

Coconut Oil

Extra virgin unrefined coconut oil is extracted by mechanical, non-heat methods from the coconut meat and coconut water.

Why is it better? You must be sure that your coconut oil is extra virgin, unrefined, otherwise it's health properties are destroyed and it may be a heart attack waiting to happen. Unrefined coconut oil is an excellent source of fat and is an antibacterial and antiviral, both topically and when eaten. Lauric acid helps the body to use the fats in coconut oil more efficiently than other fats and it also builds the immune system. Capric acid helps to protect against viruses such as HIV and sexually transmitted diseases. Research has shown that natural coconut fat in the diet leads to a normalization of body lipids, protects against alcohol damage to the liver, and improves the immune system's anti-inflammatory response.

Where do I buy it? All health food stores and most grocery stores carry coconut oil in their healthy foods department. It is extremely important that you read the label and make sure you buy unrefined coconut oil. A good coconut oil will cost you more and is worth the extra few dollars. You can also buy it on line.

How do I use it? Coconut oil also has a high smoke point so it is an excellent choice for cooking, sautéing, baking and frying. Coconut oil is the magic ingredient in our muffins, pancakes and waffles giving them a tender crisp crust and making muffins moist and fluffy. It is great for popping your own organic popcorn and in desserts. Coconut oil becomes hard at room temperature so don't refrigerate it and it does not work well in cold foods.

To quickly melt coconut oil, put it in a heat proof dish and set in a pan of boiling filtered water or in the oven at 250 degrees F.

It is also an excellent choice for deep-frying (this would be considered a treat, not a regular choice), as it has a lower smoke point and you will be less likely to burn your food. Strain it after using and store it in the refrigerator.

Buy Extra Virgin Unrefined Coconut Oil; do not buy Refined Coconut Oil.

Flax seed Oil

Flax seed oil is made from flax seeds. It must be used raw, do not cook with Flax seed oil.

Why is it better? Flax seed Oil contains omega-6 and omega-9 essential fatty acids, B vitamins, potassium, lecithin, magnesium, fiber, protein, and zinc and also provides approximately 50% more omega-3 oils than what you could get from taking fish oil. Even better,; Flax seed oil does not store in the body as fat.

Where do I buy it? All health food stores and most grocery stores carry flax seed oil in the refrigerated section of their healthy foods department. It's important to buy high-quality flax seed oil as it is prone to rancidity. Light and oxygen will slowly breakdown the essential fatty acids. Look for flax seed oil capsules (dark coated soft gels) or oil that is bottled in amber-brown bottles, as these are more resistant to the light and oxygen. Make sure you refrigerate your flax seed oil to help extend its shelf life.

Flax seed oil takes a bit of time to be absorbed into the body before the full beneficial effects begin, ranging anywhere from a few days to as many as six weeks, depending on your overall well-being.

How do I use it? Use Flax seed oil in smoothies, dressings, drizzled over veggies in place of butter. **Do not cook with Flax seed oil!**

GREAT GRAINS

Spelt Flour Products and Cereals

Spelt is an ancient form of wheat that has not been modified by hybridizing or genetic engineering. Spelt tastes like wheat with a nuttier flavor and can be used exactly like white or whole-wheat flour in recipes.

109

Why is it better? Spelt retains the original, God-given nutritional value. Summers Sprouted Flour reports Spelt to contain 50% protein and 50% starch while modern wheat, changed by man, is now 92% starch and only 8% protein (no wonder bread makes you gain weight). Spelt contains gluten, however the level of gluten is lower than in wheat. Spelt contains an enzyme that helps the body digest gluten. Some people who cannot tolerate wheat can tolerate Spelt.

Where do I buy it? Most grocery stores carry whole grain spelt flour in their health food area. You can find Spelt flour on- line. I have only found white spelt flour at Health food markets and many health food stores. You can also buy Spelt bread, cereals, cookies, crackers, pastas, and tortillas.

How do I use it? Use spelt exactly as you would regular white or whole grain wheat flour.

Quinoa (keen-wa)

Quinoa is a high fiber, high protein; alkaline seed that can be eaten raw when sprouted or used as a cooked grain much like brown rice.

Why is it better? Quinoa is a complete protein and rich in amino acids, which are the building blocks of the body. It is gluten free and wheat free and the least allergic of all grain-types. It is an excellent protein source for anyone and especially for vegan and can be used in the daily food plan in place of animal protein or in combination with other plant proteins such as beans.

Quinoa is an alkaline seed with a high in mineral content, a much lacking element in the SAD (standard American diet). Quinoa has healthy levels of iron, phosphorous, copper and zinc. It is a great source of magnesium and manganese which are important minerals for muscle function and also high in calcium, B2, vitamin E and fiber.

Besides the nutritional benefits, it is very tasty and tends to take on the flavors it is combined with, much like brown rice. NOTE: It is high in carbohydrates and calories, however, it is a good carbohydrate. Limit Quinoa consumption to no more than ½ cup per day if you are watching your weight. Quinoa is a great carbohydrate and protein for athletes and kids.

Will my kids like it? Children generally love the texture, taste and "fun" look of quinoa. When it is cooked it has a little tail, yet it is soft with a crunch and takes on any of their favorite flavors. Quinoa is one of the best grains you could feed your child. Baby should be able to start it at the same time you would add brown rice to their diet.

Where do I buy it? Most grocery stores now carry Quinoa in their health food section. You can also get it on line. Be sure to buy organic quinoa to protect you and your loved ones from pesticide-laden food.

How much should I buy? Quinoa more than doubles in quantity when cooked so bear that in mind when making a purchase.

One cup of dry Quinoa will produce at least 2 ¼ cups cooked.

How do I store it? Prepackaged Quinoa can be stored on the shelf. If you purchase from the bulk section at the grocery store keep it in an airtight container in a cool dry place. Dry, uncooked Quinoa will last approximately two months on the shelf or three to six months in the refrigerator.

How do I prepare it? Here's a great Quinoa Time Saver! I cook one pound at a time in a large pot. I love to have it available to use for different (Quinoa) recipes and store in the freezer in Zip Loc brand Baggies in 1 cup increments. When a recipe calls for Quinoa, just pull out the number of cups you need, put the baggie in the sink in some hot water for a few minutes to thaw.

How do I eat it? Try our Quinoa recipes; they are easy, full of nutrition and delicious. Find them in Chapter 15.

HEALTHY CONDIMENTS AND SEASONINGS

Better Than Bouillon Vegetarian Vegetable Base, Gluten Free

Better Than Bouillon is a healthier version of the bouillon cubes you would typically use in soups and gravies. It is manufactured by Superior Touch Products.

Why is it better? The bouillon cubes you previously bought are made up of mostly salt, MSG and a little flavor. A call to the company assured me their product has no MSG, much less salt and the majority of the flavor comes from slow cooked vegetables, reduced to a paste.

Where do I buy it? Better Than Bouillon is always available at Health food markets; you may also be able to find it at Publix and other grocery stores. You can find a dealer in your area from their website, see chapter 19. Ask your local grocery to carry it.

How do I use it? Use it any time you would use a cube or powdered bouillon or if you need richer flavor in a stir-fry, soup, bean dish or dip.

Nut Butter, Gluten Free

Nuts finely ground for use on sandwiches, in dressings and dips. A quick and easy plant based protein. Try to find raw nut butter.

Why is it better? All nuts seeds and grains contain a measure of the harmful mold, Aflatoxin. However, peanuts have the highest concentration. Almond or cashew butter is a tasty replacement for peanut butter. Use raw almond butter, roasted cashew or macadamia butter.

Where do I buy it? Most grocery stores carry different nut butters in their health food section. Read the ingredients, raw nut butters are the best choice. Nut butters like Nutella are tasty; however, they have a high amount of added sugar and should be avoided.

How do I use it? Use nut butters any time you would use peanut butter. They are delicious in salad dressings and sauces.

Braggs Amino Acids Soy Sauce Replacement

Braggs Amino Acids is a soy sauce that does not contain MSG and has a high amino acid profile.

Why is it better? No MSG or genetically modified soy products.

Where do I buy it? Most grocery stores and health food stores carry this product.

How do I use it? In recipes calling for soy sauce or when you want to give a saltier flavor without added salt. Use sparingly.

Celtic Sea Salt

Natural Celtic Sea Salts are a "moist" unrefined sea salt usually found on the coastal areas of France. The light grey, almost light purple color comes from the clay found in the salt flats. The salt is collected by hand using traditional Celtic methods.

Why is it better? Natural gray sea salts provide renewed energy, and at the same time gives higher resistance to infections and bacterial diseases. Natural Celtic Sea Salts are the gentlest alkaline forming substance known.

"Many illnesses are caused or exacerbated by trace-mineral deficiencies. These can be avoided by the liberal use of Celtic Sea Salt® in your cooking and the complete avoidance of all other salts, all of which contain only pure sodium chloride." Dr. Thomas S. Cowan, M.D

Where do I buy it? You can find it at Health food market and in the health food section at most grocery stores. You can also buy it on –line.

How do I use it? You may buy it in the fine ground form, or in crystals, which may be ground in a mortar. Celtic Sea Salt is moist, not dry like your typical table salt. Use it as you would salt, sparingly in your everyday food.

Tahini, Gluten Free

Tahini is ground sesame paste, similar to nut butter. You can make it yourself or purchase it pre-made.

Why is it better? There are many good reasons to use Tahini and Sesame seeds in general. Sesame seeds are extremely high in calcium, good fat and have higher amino acid profile than other plant proteins such as beans. They also contain lignans, an excellent antioxidant. Sesame seeds are known to lower cholesterol, relieve constipation and remove worms from the intestinal tract. They aid digestion and stimulate blood circulation and benefit the nervous system.

Where do I buy it? You can make your own Tahini by grinding sesame seeds in a magic bullet or high-speed blender or you can purchase it at and most health food stores. Store it in the refrigerator after you open it and use it regularly as it will go rancid after a few months.

How do I use it? Tahini can be used in place of peanut butter in recipes. It is usually called for in Middle Eastern recipes such as baba ghanoush, hummus and halvah. It is also used in salad dressing recipes and sauces.

Grape Seed Veganaise

A vegan (vegetarian, no animal products) mayonnaise made with Grape seed oil.

Why is it better? Grape seed Veganaise has an excellent flavor. Grape seed oil is known to lower cholesterol. It has a very small amount of soy, which is the predominant ingredient in other vegan mayonnaise. It is also free of harmful additives and preservatives.

Where do I buy it? Grape seed Veganaise is available at Health food market, some health food stores and on-line. It is in the refrigerated section.

How do I use it? Use it in place of mayonnaise in salad dressings, dips, and spreads, on sandwiches and in place of buttermilk in baked goods.

BETTER DAIRY CHOICES

Raw Grass Fed Cheese & Dairy Products

Grass Fed, Raw milk products such as cheese, milk, yogurt, sour cream and butter come from cows raised on organic pasture grass. The flavor is unbelievable. You actually taste the flavor of the food right away so you don't need as much. **Ghee** is clarified butter, the butterfat without the milk solids. Buy it at most groceries in the butter section...important, only use organic.

Why is it better? The food enzymes are intact to help your body digest the dairy products. Raw, grass-fed dairy products are high in the healthy omega-3 fatty acids so severely lacking in most people's diets. This translates to a better-balanced ratio of omega 6 to omega 3 in your diet, which has been shown to lower the risk of cancer, heart disease, diabetes, obesity, and mental disorders. A small piece of raw cheese goes a long way, this gives flavor with less calories. Raw cheese is made from unpasteurized, raw milk.

Where do I buy it? (Raw Milk Products) Some grocery stores carry raw cheese in the refrigerated part of their health food section or deli. You can also find raw cheese on line, at Health food market and in specialty shops. It will specifically say "made from raw milk" or "made from unpasteurized milk" on the package or in the Ingredients. Other items made from unpasteurized milk, such as milk to drink, raw butter, sour cream and yogurt must be purchased directly from the farmer. Go to www.localharvest.org and type in "raw milk" for a supplier near you.

How do I use it? Raw milk, butter, yogurt, cream and sour cream may be used in exact quantities to replace pasteurized milk products. Use raw cheese just like you would any other cheeses but in smaller amounts. The flavor is powerful so you can have lots of flavor and less fat and calories.

What about yogurt? Read the ingredients on your yogurt label. Jordan Rubin and David Brascoe, MD, in their book **Restoring Your Digestive Health** cite research that the bacteria "s.thermophilus" found in almost all commercially produced yogurts is known to stimulate auto immune disease. Avoid yogurt with "s.thermophilus" ingredient. There is an easy yogurt recipe in Chapter 11. Erivan yogurt is made from unpasteurized milk and only contains the acidophilus bacteria, proven to be beneficial. It can be purchased at Health food market or check their website for a local source.

WHAT TO BUY ORGANIC

There are several types of organic foods you can purchase; **Prepared Organic Foods** such as cereals, breads, salad dressings, canned and frozen foods. **Fresh produce** and **Naturally Raised Animal and Dairy products**.

If you choose to use prepared foods you should buy and eat as much organic as possible. Typically, true organic prepared foods do not have harmful additives, dyes, preservatives, hormones and antibiotics.

That said, it is important to read the ingredients on any product to be sure it contains only good food. Non-organic foods are laden with harmful chemical preservatives and additives, trans Fats, excessive sugars, and genetically modified products, especially oils.

Watch all products, even at health food stores for genetically modified oils; Soybean oil, Canola Oil, Cottonseed Oil and Corn oil. If a product is certified organic it cannot contain genetically modified ingredients. Most packaging will state "NON-GMO" or "NON-GE" if they do not use genetically modified oils.

<< *You will find a credit card sized "what to buy organic" list to cut out and keep in your wallet with the pull out pantry and shopping lists at the end of the book.* >>

Organic Produce
You may not always find and possibly cannot afford to buy all organic veggies and fruits.

Many people do not understand the value of organic foods and believe it is a marketing hoax. You will read articles claiming no difference between organic fruits and vegetables and non-organic.

Studies have shown organic foods contain higher levels of minerals; up to 2,000 times that of non-organic foods. It is virtually impossible to eat only organic foods, however, do a "taste test" and compare the flavor of organic and non-organic produce. You will likely find the organic more flavorful, unless, however, you just picked something fresh from your own garden!

When you must buy non-organic foods you will get better value and nutrients from local growers at your local farmers market. Local produce is usually allowed to ripen longer, allowing more nutrients to develop and be released in the food. Produce shipped long distances, for instance from foreign countries or coast to coast in the United States are picked very early, gassed to prevent quick ripening and then shipped to you. Local is ALWAYS a better choice. Find local growers at http://www.localharvest.org

Naturally Raised Animal and Dairy Products
We follow Dr. Joel Fuhrman's recommended amount animal protein limiting intake to less than 12 ounces per week. If your budget only allows you to choose organic produce or organic meats, start with the meat. The greatest dangers to your health are in the hamburgers, chicken nuggets and fish fillets you eat every day.

Meats, eggs, fish, cheeses and milk products purchased from restaurants, fast food joints, frozen home delivery services, and your regular super market or grocery store are made from animals raised on foods they were not created to eat. The animals are in unsanitary and inhumane conditions, they must be pumped full of pharmaceutical drugs to be kept alive and are not processed in ways that promote health. A great movie to watch to learn more about the handling of commercially grown meat is "FOOD INC", released in 2009. You can find it on line at www.foodincmovie.com, everyone over twelve years of age in your family should watch this movie.

DAIRY: Only buy organic milk, butter, cheese, ice cream, yogurt, etc. Raw cheese, raw butter, raw milk made .from unpasteurized milk is the best. If you have questions about raw milk check out the Weston Price website, www.realmilk.com. They address everything from health and safety issues to why raw milk products are more healthful. Limit your consumption of dairy products because it is acid forming and should be included in the "12 ounces or less per week" guideline.

Whey protein powders come from cows. Only buy organic whey protein powder; free from rBGH

RED MEAT: Beef, Bison, Lamb, Pork. Only buy "naturally grown" without antibiotics and hormones and GRASS FED. All animals that give us red meat were created to eat grass, not corn, oats and rye. Grass fed meat is becoming increasingly more available and you can find a local grower at www.localharvest.org. We do not eat pork at all.

POULTRY: Only buy "naturally grown" without antibiotics and hormones and FREE RANGE or PASTURED.

EGGS: Buy your eggs from a local grower, there are plenty around, even in the city you can find them at the Farmer's Market. Health food markets usually carries locally grown eggs as well.

PORK: Pork is not healthy meat in any way shape or form. Pigs are typically not fed good food, there are grass fed pigs which would produce a better quality of meat, however, pork in any form, whether ham, bacon, sausage, pork chops, pork roast or any other form you might eat, is a toxic meat.

"Recent research indicates the "other white meat" is a passageway for a number of serious illnesses, which can jump from animals to human hosts. And the intensive, factory farm conditions by which most pigs are raised increases the risk and acts as an incubator for bacteria. There's also proof, for the first time, that using antibiotics to treat pigs can lead to outbreaks of dangerous human diseases like salmonella."
http://www.organicconsumers.org/toxic/porkfilth.cfm

FISH: WILD CAUGHT, Cold Water Fish Only! The same problems that exist in beef and chicken growing factories exist in fish growing factories. Shellfish and crustaceans are the vacuum cleaners of the water, and full of toxins.

Save Money on Your Food Budget

The healthiest and most economical proteins you can eat are plant proteins. Beans are a great weight loss food and the perfect blend of carbohydrates, and protein containing little to no fat! Dr. Joel Fuhrman, <u>Eat</u> <u>To</u> <u>Live</u> recommends everyone have a minimum of 1 cup of cooked beans per day.

If you compare the fact that one pound of beans will usually cost less than $1.50 to the fact that one pound of grass-fed or pastured animal protein ranges in cost from $3 to $21 per pound, you might be encouraged to know that in the long run, one pound of healthy, fibrous beans can feed two people for at least a week.

Beans are extremely flavorful and versatile so we recommend cooking several different types of beans to discover which ones you like best and which ways you prefer to prepare them. Try making hummus from black beans or garbanzos and use it as a spread for sandwiches or as a dip. Also bean soups such as lentil soup are delicious. Add beans to your vegetable soup. Make a salad topping with beans, salsa and avocado. Make your own veggie burgers with beans. See chapter 15 for delicious bean recipes. You can use canned beans, rather than cooking dry beans, this will increase the cost as you should only use organic canned beans.

Another delicious and economical form of plant protein is nuts and seeds such as almonds, sunflower seeds and pumpkin seeds. Eat a handful of soaked nuts, seeds or a couple of tablespoons of nut butter instead of animal protein or beans a few times a week.

More Ways To Save Money On Groceries
Buy conventionally and locally grown produce that have low pesticide levels (see "what to buy organic" at the end of the book) and only buy organic items on the high pesticide list. If you have a compromised immune system, like cancer or an autoimmune disease, all your food should be organic.

Make your own food. The biggest portion of a high food bill is processed foods. If you are going to eat well you will either spend time preparing your food or spend money paying for pre-made food. Use the bulk aisle at Whole Foods or join a natural foods coop. You can buy just the amount you need or purchase staples on line.

In Their Own Words

While the detox was not fun at first, it was empowering and exhilarating after the first few rough spots. During the first month my bad cholesterol dropped over 50% and my good increased 3 times. When my doctor did the blood work again six weeks after the reflux ordeal he sent me a note saying that this report was a grand slam!!! He had not seen such a radical reduction in such a short time. My wife also added more strength and energy to her life as well as reducing body fat. (She also was not overweight.)

Over the course of the last 12 months I have found those foods that I can re-enter into my eating patterns. My health has never been better ... I am still actively engaged in my process and have been able to find the balance in my food choices which I know has extended my physical well being. Simply stated, I am better. I go back for a scan in June and for my next round of blood work, and am eager to receive the results.

This process is a gift ... all that is required is the willingness to be willing to change! As it is said in one fellowship ... "It works if you work it." And I would add, if you are sick and tired of being sick and tired. I was! RD, M, 50+ Our Note: Cholesterol dropped 100 points in 28-days..

"I have tested my ph for years and it has always been very acidic. After the first week of detox, I lost 8 pounds and brought my body pH up *to 7, where it should be. It has never been that high! The pain I lived with daily is gone and I feel like a new person." VM, F, 52 (28-day weight loss 15 pounds). Our Note: a normal pH for human blood is 7.4 and urine is 6.*

CHAPTER 7   EATING FOR BALANCE

How many diets have you tried over the years? Many Americans are on a continual diet of some type. High Protein, Low Protein, Low Carb, Low Fat, Low Sugar, the list goes on. Most popular diets, especially the ones that sell you prepackaged foods, are based on dead, low nutrient food. You may lose weight but you won't necessarily be healthy.

The alkaline diet is the best way to promote health in your body. It involves reducing the acid forming foods in your every day diet and increasing the alkaline foods, which balance body chemistry. A balanced alkaline diet reduces inflammation, which is the root of many diseases. Research has shown that degenerative diseases such as Type 2 Diabetes cannot survive in a body that is in a true alkaline state.

Many books have been written on the Alkaline Diet. You can check the acidity of your own body with ph paper but honestly, if you are currently eating the Standard American Diet (S.A.D.) you are definitely eating an acidic diet and so your body is most likely in an acid state. The alkaline diet is easy, eat mostly fresh fruits and vegetables, reduce or eliminate acid forming foods, reverse negative thinking and your body should become alkaline. A list of acid forming foods follows.

123

Alkaline Balanced Whole Food Plan

15% Fresh Fruit

35% Raw
Veggies

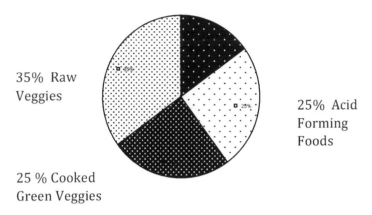

25% Acid
Forming
Foods

25 % Cooked
Green Veggies

The above graph shows what your daily food intake should look like as defined by Alkaline Diet expert, Dr. Ted M. Morter, Jr., M.A. author of **Health and Wellness, Your Absolute Quintessential, All You Wanted To Know Guide**. To emphasize the importance of eating less acid forming foods and more alkaline forming foods, Dr. Morter states:

"Unprotected sensitive tissue that is designed to carry alkaline materials is defenseless against acid substances."

Eat More Fresh Veggies and Less Meats of All Kinds

Dr. Joel Fuhrman, MD, in his book Eat To Live suggests you eat at least 1 cup of beans per day and 1 ½ to 2 pounds of vegetables per day. Limit animal proteins to 2-4 ounces per day, less than 12 ounces per week.

One to two and a half pounds sounds like a lot of veggies, I know, however, if you drink 1-8 ounce glass of fresh carrot juice you have already consumed 1 lb of raw carrots, a great way to get your veggies in. Add 4 handfuls of fresh leafy greens, 2 to lunch and 2 to dinner, some cooked veggies and some colorful veggies on with your leafy greens and you easily have the two pounds suggested by Dr. Fuhrman. You will get to the point where you want these veggies, even if you think you don't like veggies now!

Learn the Alkaline Diet for life in our program My Busy Healthy Life; more info on our website, www.thewellnessworkshop.org. Click the "Start Here" button.

ALKALINE DIET

Eat 15% Raw Fruit Daily
Fruit is alkalizing and cleansing. Enjoy fresh fruit in the morning. Try eating only juicy raw fruits until after your first BM of the day. Many times people who are constipated report this alleviates their constipation after just a few days.

<< Acid Forming Foods: Limit to 25% daily - Animal Proteins, Dairy products, Beans and Legumes, Grains, Sugar, Caffeine, Nuts and Seeds (quinoa and almonds are alkaline) >>

Limit These Acid Forming Foods to 25%
The foods in the box cause acid to form in your body. Your body will need to neutralize the acid with valuable minerals. Degenerative diseases such as cancer and diabetes flourish in an acid environment.

Eat 25% Cooked Green Veggies Daily
Some of the vitamins in greens are better absorbed by lightly cooking; sauté or steam. Only eat spinach raw and uncooked.

Eat 35% Raw Veggies Daily
Vegetables are healing and alkalizing. Everyone should get four handfuls of leafy greens per day and a variety of other colorful veggies. It is especially important for athletes to maintain an alkaline balanced diet. Each year the news

reports athletes' young and old who seemed healthy but suddenly die in the midst of competition, such as runners at the end of a marathon, football and soccer players in the midst of a game. On page 67 of his book, Dr. Ted Morter explains:

"The only time when <u>naturally produced</u> acid (produced by the body) may become a health threat is when acid from strenuous exercise tops off excess acid from food. Joggers, professional athletes and other who exercise a lot are at risk if their systems have already reached the maximum tolerable limits of dietary acid build-up. If they are already acidotic, when they exercise, acid is generated faster than the body can get rid of it. If they can live long enough to pant, they'll survive. If they can't, they don't."

An Alkaline Food Day
Fresh veggie juice in place of coffee.

Breakfast
Fresh pineapple, strawberries and blueberries with half cup homemade organic yogurt.

Snack
15 raw , soaked almonds.

Lunch
2 handfuls of leafy greens with shredded carrot, radish, green onion, broccoli, and cucumber, 2 ounces of grilled chicken or half cup 3 Bean salad topped with some crunchy quinoa.

Snack
Fresh veggie juice or an apple with 2 Tablespoons raw almond butter.

Dinner

2 handfuls of leafy greens with a variety of veggies and your favorite homemade dressing, Asian stir fry and quinoa or brown rice.

Snack

Barney Smoothie or Nutty Buddy Almond Butter Balls.

Water
Half your body weight in ounces of water every day.

Are You Looking For Permanent Life Change?

My Busy Healthy Life, our 4 month web-based coaching program, walks you step by step from drinking water, completing a 28-day cleanse, learning to listen to your body and finally creating an alkaline food plan that works in your real life. For more info on My Busy Healthy Life go to our website, www.thewellnessworkshop.org and click the "Start Here" button.

In Their Own Words

"When I first began my detox journey, (I had been on a pre-packaged weight loss program for almost a year) I was exhausted, had little energy, was discouraged with the inability to lose weight, and my allergies symptoms were over-active.

The best personal investment I made was enrolling in the Give Your Body A Break Detox. I received Personal coaching about how to avoid "dead" food and recipe demonstrations throughout my detox period made my success in the program possible.

I had restored energy and increased focus. I defeated the weight plateau barrier and my allergy symptoms essentially disappeared. The changes to my skin were amazing--no one ever complains about looking younger! I am a believer and continue to endorse the program. RH, F, 50+

127

These are based on the alkaline balance food circle. There are a few recipes that use eggs. To be completely vegan use Enr-g Egg Substitute or 2 Tablespoons ground flax seed mixed with 4 Tablespoons filtered water and let sit for 10 minutes before using.

For optimal health drink a minimum of 16 ounces up to 32 ounces of fresh, raw veggie juice each day; breakfast, morning and afternoon snack. Drink more juice if you are fighting disease. Always drink half your body weight in filtered water.

Quick Breakfast Ideas
16 ounces freshly made vegetable juice.

Eat your 15% fruit here – fruit only until BM in the AM.

After BM have a sprouted grain product or sprouted cereal product with alternative milk such as almond milk, hemp milk or goats milk.

Protein Shake (no soy) We like Garden of Life Raw Protein or Jay Robb's unflavored Whey, rBGH free.

Quick Lunches & Dinners
35% Raw Veggies
Salad with 2 handfuls of greens or romaine, top with a variety of veggies and your favorite beans.

And choose one
Phil's Kitchen Sink Soup
Green Goddess Sandwich with sprouted grain bread
Rice Paper Wraps

Mexican Meal

Even the pickiest eater will enjoy any of these Mexican entrees. They are familiar flavors and textures made with healthier ingredients. The easiest recipe is Three Bean Chili. The most complicated but best comfort food is Chili Relleno Casserole.

My favorite is Quinoa Stuffed Peppers and the Chili Relleno Casserole.

THINGS YOU CAN DO AHEAD
Chop and sauté veggies, cook Quinoa, make spelt tortillas, grate cheese and assemble the end product.
Make slaw and salads, cook beans in crock-pot, make Quinoa Stuffed Peppers, 3 Bean Chili and organic corn bread and put in freezer for later.

Make pico de gallo and guacamole up to 3 days in advance. Buy organic corn chips.

==

Strawberry Lemonade

STARTERS & SIDES

Spinach or Romaine Salad with Herb Vinaigrette

Refried beans

Pico de Gallo

Guacamole

Organic corn chips

CHOOSE ONE ENTRÉE

Veggie Fajitas

Spinach Enchiladas

129

Quinoa Stuffed Peppers

Three Bean Chili with Organic Corn Muffins

Bean Burritos with home made Spelt Tortillas

===

Faux Crab Cakes Meal

I love crab cakes, however, I don't eat crab because it is an extremely toxic food. These have the flavors and textures of wonderful crab cakes without the toxicity. They can be made ahead and frozen.

THINGS YOU CAN DO AHEAD
Bake spaghetti squash, freeze in zip loc bags for later use; some for crab cakes, some for spaghetti. Make Roasted Red Pepper Dressing, and Green Goddess Dressing up to 3 days prior.

===

Apple Lemonade

FAUX CRAB CAKES

Spinach salad with veggies tossed in Green Goddess Dressing

Veggie tray with Green Goddess dressing

Green Beans sautéed with garlic and basil

Faux "Crab" Cakes drizzled with Roasted Red Pepper Dressing

===

Asian Meal

My favorite everyday lunch is the Asian Sprout Salad. I love to take the Sushi Salad to dinner parties where it is promptly devoured and receives lots of ooohhhs and aaaahs.

ASIAN

Asian Cabbage Salad

Quinoa

Orange Ginger Stir Fry

Sushi Salad

DESSERT

Coconut Ice Cream drizzled with lime zest and honey

===

Italian Meal

Both of these menus are personal favorites. Your family and friends will enjoy them as well. They can easily be made ahead and frozen for up to one month. Prepare a double batch, serve one and freeze one!

Spaghetti Primavera: Precook Squash and freeze in one-cup portions in zip loc Baggies. Cut veggies for sauce and salad and make salad dressing and sauce up to 3 days in advance. You can also use a prepared sauce, we like Newman's Organics or Muir Glen.

Zucchini Lasagna: Make Zucchini Lasagna recipe, freeze. Make spinach pesto made with raw cheese. Freeze.

Homemade Ice Cream and Grandma Davises Spelt Chocolate Chip Cookies make a great dessert!

131

==

Harvest Cocktail

SPAGHETTI PRIMAVERA

*Large Italian Vegetable Salad tossed in Robb's Balsamic
Vinaigrette*

Spaghetti Squash with Primavera sauce

ZUCCHINI LASAGNE

*Romaine salad with Tomatoes, red onion and Mushrooms
tossed in Roasted Garlic Vinaigrette*

Zucchini Lasagna

Toasted sprouted sourdough bread with Spinach

==

Pizza Meal

When we first detoxed Pizza was a once a month treat for
me, but it had to be a REALLY good pizza. I learned to make
my own and really enjoy it. All the pizza choices are
delicious and much healthier than frozen or restaurant
pizzas.

THINGS YOU CAN DO AHEAD

Pizza Crust: Prebake Homemade Spelt Pizza crust. Cut up
veggies for veggie tray or salad and pizza toppings. Make
Real Ranch Dressing. Assemble pizza just prior to baking.

Prebaked crusts save time, try a sprouted one like the Alvarado Street bakery.

The zucchini crust pizza is yummy and you can make extra to eat for lunches.

===

Wally-ade

PIZZA NIGHT

Raw Veggie Tray

Fresh Garden Salad with Real Ranch Dressing

CHOOSE PIZZA

Homemade Spelt Pizza with Raw Cheese and Veggie Toppings

Quick Flat Bread Pizza

Alvarado Street Sprouted Pizza Crust with your favorite toppings

Zucchini Crust Pizza

DESSERT

Homemade Ice Cream

Grandma Davis' Oatmeal Chocolate Chip Cookies

===

CHAPTER 8   DETOX

OUR "GIVE YOUR BODY A BREAK" 28-DAY DETOX

In the first chapter of this book I told my story. My health journey started with a body detox program that lasted 21-days. In those 21-days I was able to lose 16 pounds and all of my medical conditions. It has been clinically proven that the body responds in 21 day increments, thus most natural health programs take place over a 21-day period of time. We do our program over a 28-day period to allow people to first eliminate their addictive foods, alcohol, caffeine and sugar.

Most people will benefit from a body detox program. Consult with a trained, licensed medical professional on all matters pertaining to your health.

UPDATE NOTE: The detox (cleanse) in this book is excellent for people who do not mind making their own food or their own juices. If you have a very busy life and/or do not like to make your own food I suggest our plan for busy people, My Busy Healthy Life that takes just a few minutes of preparation a day. Find more information on My Busy Healthy Life at our website, www.thewellnessworkshop.org.

Help Your Body Detox on a Daily Basis
Your body was created to detoxify (eliminate toxins) on a daily basis. These are the things you can do to help your body do its job and keep you healthy.

√ Drink ½ your body weight in ounces of filtered water
√ Get at least 8 hours of sleep
√ Get 15-30 minutes of sunshine- no sunscreen-daily
√ Move your body 30 minutes per day minimum
√ Eat 65-75% of your daily food as raw fruits & veggies
√ Completely Eliminate refined sugar, hydrogenated oils and chemicals (especially artificial sweeteners)
√ Limit alcohol to less than two times per week

What Is A Body Detox Program?
Detoxifying the body has been practiced by cultures worldwide for thousands of years. Detoxing became a fad since 1989 when the American Cancer Research Center released its findings that the body's natural ability to detoxify affects the occurrence of disease. (The Detox Revolution, Thomas J. Slaga, PhD.)

Many people go to the health food store and buy a "box detox" that promises more energy, less aches and pains and rapid weight loss. These same people generally quit within the first 3-5 days due to the increase in their aches and pains and even flu-like symptoms as the body does its job of eliminating toxins. Those who are successful in completing the prescribed program do feel an increase in energy, less aches and pains and weight loss. However, if they don't change the food they are eating and their lifestyle they quickly become toxic again and the benefits were short lived.

Maca

Maca Shooters. Maca is a root vegetable from Peru known to rebuild weak organs. It is especially helpful for the adrenal glands to increase stamina and male and female reproductive systems. It can help with infertility and low libido in both men and women. A bag of Maca at Health food markets at this writing costs approximately $25.00, however, it will last one person many months as you use only 1 teaspoon per day.

Flax Seed And Hemp Seeds In Your Morning Smoothies

Flax seeds are rich in Alpha Linoleic Acid, an important form of Omega 3 fat. 2 Tablespoons of flax seed, ground and uncooked are attributed with excellent anti-inflammatory properties. They are also known to protect bone health, protect the body from cancer, diabetes, and heart disease. Prevent and control high blood pressure and lower blood pressure in men with high cholesterol. Flax seeds are rich in fiber. Studies have shown them to slow the growth of prostate cancer and be effective in reducing the risk of breast cancer. They have also been shown to fend off dry eyes and hot flashes.

Hemp seeds. In his book Fats that Heal, Fats that Kill, Udo Erasmus, © Alive Books, December 1993 states "A pound of hemp seed would provide all the protein, essential fatty acids and dietary fiber necessary for human survival for two weeks. The protein in hemp contains all eight amino acids essential to life and is easily digested. For this reason it is used in many parts of the world for treating malnourishment."

Digestive Enzymes

Digestive Enzymes are recommended for most Americans. Our diet of mostly cooked foods has drastically compromised our body's supply of digestive enzymes, evidenced by the fact that according to Consumer Reports, in 2008 the "purple pill" used for poor digestion, was the second most used drug in America.

We use digestive enzymes when we eat cooked foods and plant and animal proteins. We like Garden of Life Ultra Omegazyme. Some people may also need to add a supplement of hydrochloric acid (HCL), especially those over 50 years of age as the body reduces production of hydrochloric acid as we age.

Proteolytic Enzymes (Protease).

These enzymes help to reduce inflammation, increase blood flow, break down proteins from toxins and reduce withdrawal symptoms when eliminating caffeine, alcohol and sugar. Garden of Life Wobenzyme or Transformation Enzymes Protease 375K are excellent choices.

"Living" High-Count Probiotics

This explanation is from the website of Udo's Choice probiotics.

What are probiotics? "The human gastrointestinal tract is home to more than 400 types of probiotics (i.e., "friendly" bowel bacteria, gut microorganisms, or intestinal flora). In fact, more probiotics live in a person's mouth than there have ever been human beings on this Earth.

These "friendly" microorganisms protect the GI tract (from mouth to anus) and keep us healthy by protecting us from "unfriendly" microorganisms such as bacteria, yeasts, and fungi that cause disease. They also improve immune system function, and have other health benefits."

Babies receive probiotics at birth from the mother's birth canal. Recent practices of having mothers take an antibiotic week s before birth may compromise babies' immune system and their ability to digest food. Babies who are delivered C-section may also miss these vital microorganisms. For some good information on probiotics, check out the website http://www.udoerasmus.com/products/probiotics_en.htm.

Cleansing Your Organs

There are other liver, kidney and colon supplements you can add to your detox, check with your local health food store for their recommendations. Two companies we trust are Garden of Life and Udo's Choice, both have several cleansing products. We use Garden of Life's **Raw Cleanse** for a periodic, 10 day cleanse once a year. A cleanse is also beneficial after a prolonged illness or medication and after vacations where food has not been optimal.

Give your Body a Break So It Can Do Its Job

Your body was created to detox on a daily basis. The food you eat and the lifestyle you live determine how your body deals with toxins. Our detox program is designed to support your body's own detoxification system with the food it needs and give you an awareness of toxic foods and habits that you can change or eliminate to keep from becoming toxic all over again.

Included in this book is our 28-day, *Give Your Body A Break* Detox plan. Many people, like me, have completely eliminated chronic physical conditions like Type 2 Diabetes, Irritable Bowel Syndrome, Eczema, Psoriasis, High Blood Pressure, High Cholesterol, Arthritis, Depression and a host of other physical complaints that are actually caused by eating toxic foods, thinking toxic thoughts and not giving your body the food and filtered water it needs to function.

During the detox you eliminate the 7 offending foods for 28-days and then reintroduce them slowly, one at a time for 3 days at a time. As you add the foods back in and listen to your body, it will let you know if the food is not good for you. You will find more information on the 7 Offending Foods in Chapter 3.

The changes are simple, although they are not easy because you are going against the American culture of food and lifestyle.

You will also find our Detox, ETC life plan, which stands for Detox one day per week and then the rest of the week, Eat, Treat and Celebrate.

WEEKLY MEAL PLANS WE USE FOR A 28-DAY DETOX

DAYS 1-7 REDUCE TO ELIMINATE

In your first week of detox you must eliminate addictive foods. Avoid alcohol, caffeine and sugar completely for 28 days.

<< *DAYS 1-7:* REDUCE TO ELIMINATE ADDICTIVE FOODS – ALCOHOL, CAFFEINE, SUGAR & NON-SUGAR SWEETENERS. >>

The best way to accomplish this is by reducing the amount you use each day until it is completely eliminated. We call this the "reduce to eliminate" week. Use half as much each day until you are completely off these three foods.

You may experience withdrawal symptoms as you reduce to eliminate alcohol, caffeine or sugar, typically headaches, body aches, tiredness. Plan to have the option to stay home and rest during this time and be sure to drink a lot of filtered water, tea, and broth. People who drink large amounts of diet sodas or use large amounts of artificial sweeteners may experience flu-like symptoms on day 5; these normally involve vomiting, diarrhea, headache, body ache and last approximately 24 hours. Please remember to consult your health care provider for all matters pertaining to your health.

Drink Water
You will also need to start drinking more filtered water, working up to half your body weight in ounces of filtered water. If you weigh 200 pounds, you would need to drink 100 ounces of filtered water daily. Buy filtered, alkaline water. Deer Park Spring water is one of the more alkaline grocery store brands. If you are drinking at least 16 ounces of fresh juice per day you can use distilled filtered water, if not use filtered spring water. See Chapter 19 for resources.

FOOD DAYS 1-7

Food changes in Week 1 are very simple, eat whatever you like as you are getting off your addictive foods but add in some raw fruits and veggies.

**Breakfast: ADD 1 raw fruit to your typical breakfast.
Lunch & Dinner: ADD 1 raw vegetable to your typical lunch and dinner.**

In Their Own Words
"I was tired, over weight, and had severe headaches and migraines daily. I thought my eating was ok....I ate cereal or toast for breakfast and fast food for lunch....dinner was pastas or whatever we felt like eating as a big family dinner.   And boy did I ever snack afterwards!

My detox lasted about 1 month. I ate raw fruits and veggies, and my beverage was only water. I increased my water intake by ½ bottle per 30 minutes during my workday. I cut out my unhealthy snacking too. Within 10 days I started to feel better, less headaches and more energy!

Within 6 months of my new life style, I have lost more than 30 pounds! My daily headaches have decreased to only once a week or so, because of I've figured out what foods caused them – milk products; chemicals and yeast products were giving me side effects.

My new life style has positively impacted all areas of my life from family, job to social. I am now more engaged in the people in my life, and happier everywhere I go during my day because I feel better and I have more energy to fuel me throughout my day! SM, M, 40+

===

REDUCE TO ELIMINATE

Alcohol, Caffeine, Sugar

INCREASE WATER

Drink half your body weight in ounces of filtered water.

RAW FOOD

Add 1 raw fruit to breakfast.

Add 1 raw vegetable to lunch.

Add 1 raw vegetable to dinner.

PROTEOLYC ENZYMES

As Directed

===

REDUCE TO ELIMINATE ADDICTIVE FOODS

Replace Alcohol *with filtered water or an occasional mineral water.*

Replace Caffeine *with Green Tea. Try a Green Tea Miso with Stevia or an herbal tea.*

Replace Sugar *with yummy, juicy fresh fruit when you would normally reach for cookies, candy or ice cream. Make sure fruit is always available.*

Water, Water, Water!
Half your body weight in ounces per day, no exceptions!

Normal detox reactions would be flu-like symptoms such as headaches, achiness and nausea, which should pass within 24 hours. Proteolytic Enzymes may help with these symptoms.

Severe pain, excessive vomiting, diarrhea, dry heaves are not typical.

===

100% RAW DAYS

MORNING

32 ounces warm water juice of 1 lemon

Proteolytic Enzyme

Probiotic

Antioxidant Juice

Maca Shooter

143

Hemp & Flax Smoothie

LUNCH & DINNER

2 handfuls leafy greens w/ vinaigrette dressing

Variety of raw veggies

Side salad

Beans, Nuts, Seeds

TREAT

Nutty Buddy Almond Butter Balls

==

Always consult with your licensed health professional on all matters pertaining to your health.

DAYS 8-10 –

100% RAW VEGGIES & FRUITS & COOKED PROTEINS

ELIMINATE
> Alcohol
> Caffeine
> Chemicals
> Dairy
> Grains
> Sugar
> Limit Animal Protein to 12 ounces per week

Important!
Drink juice on an empty stomach, with only water and wait 20 minutes eating.

Limit fruit to 3 per day, including smoothies.

Water Half your body weight in ounces per day, no exceptions!

100% Raw Days Menu Ideas

Protein – Choose 1 per lunch and dinner

1 ounce Almonds, Sunflower Seeds, Pumpkin Seeds, Pecans

1cup beans per day, minimum at lunch or dinner

Protein shakes that are OK: Standard Process SP Complete, Jay Robb's with Stevia and Garden of Life Perfect Meal or Raw Protein

2-3 ounces organic eggs, fish, red meat, chicken, turkey

Dressing Choice

Robb's Italian Dressing

Dijon Mustard Vinaigrette

Herb dressing

Side Salad Choice

3-Minute Salad

Aunt Celeste's Kale Salad

Asian Broccoli Slaw

Protein Choice

Black Bean Salsa Salad

3 Bean Salad

Protein Shake

Sample Lunch
Leafy Green Salad with Herb dressing, ½ cup Aunt Celeste's
Kale Salad, 1 cup 3 Minute Salad, ½ cup 3-Bean Salad

Sample Dinner
Leafy Green Salad with Dijon Mustard Vinaigrette, Butter
Bean Hummus with Carrot & Celery Sticks, ½ cup Black Bean
Salsa and Guacamole

For Crunch on your salad or soup (in place of croutons and
bacon bits) try Crunchy Quinoa or Pumpkin Seed Crunch.

Sample Treat
2 Nutty Buddy Almond Butter Balls

In Their Own Words

*"I identified with many of the issues around a lack of digestive
enzymes, but had put it down to being overweight, being
menopausal, being stressed out. At my first consultation, I
learned that my binge eating was probably due to the fact that
I was not receiving the nutrition from the food that I was
consuming. My body lacks digestive enzymes, so even though I
was eating ever-increasing amounts I was constantly hungry,
constantly thinking about food.*

*I immediately started taking digestive enzymes with every
meal. The enzymes now allow my body to digest the food
properly and extract the nutrients from the food. As a result,
all desire for binge eating has gone. My aches and pains, too,
have all but completely disappeared; the pain had been caused
by inflammation from the toxins in the food I had been
consuming over the years. Best of all, I've dropped two dress
sizes! Better than best of all, I am continuing with the
program; it's not a "diet" that has an end date, it's now become
a way of life". JS, F, 50+*

DAYS 11-28

WE CALL THESE THE 75/25 DAYS. COOK 25% OF YOUR VEGGIES IF YOU PREFER.

75% RAW VEGGIES & FRUIT

25% COOKED VEGGIES

COOKED PROTEINS

NUTS & SEEDS

ELIMINATE
    Alcohol
    Caffeine
    Chemicals
    Dairy
    Grains
    Sugar

    Limit Animal Protein to 12 ounces per week

Important!
Drink Juice on empty stomach. 3 fruits/day. **Water!**

===

75/25 DAYS

MORNING

32 ounces warm water with juice of 1 lemon

Proteolytic Enzyme

Probiotic

Antioxidant Juice

147

Maca Shooter

MID MORNING & AFTERNOON SNACK

Barney Hemp & Flax Smoothie

LUNCH & DINNER

2 handfuls leafy greens w/ vinaigrette dressing

Variety of raw veggies, 25% cooked veggies

Side salad

Beans, Nuts, Seeds

TREAT

Baked Apple

==

75/25 Days Menu Ideas

Dressing Choice

Cherry Balsamic Vinaigrette

Roasted Garlic Dressing

Herb Dressing

Side Choice

Quick Asian Broccoli Salad

Garlicky Kale Salad

Quinoa Tabooli

Protein Choice

Vegetarian Bean Burgers

Sweet & Spicy Pecans

Add Beans and Quinoa to Phil's Kitchen Sink Soup

Cooked Veggies

Phil's Kitchen Sink Soup

Treat

Raw Peach Cobbler

Sample Lunch or Dinner

Harvest Time Green Salad with Cherry Balsamic Vinaigrette, Garlicky Kale Salad and Phil's Kitchen Sink Soup.

Missing Croutons? Try Crunchy Quinoa on Salad or in soup.

More 75/25 Menu Ideas

Dressing Choice
Orange Ginger Vinaigrette

Lime Vinaigrette

Roasted Red Pepper Dressing

Side Choice
Jicama Salad

Asian Bean Sprout Salad

Rice Paper Wraps

Protein Choice
Roasted Red Pepper Humus

3 Bean Chili

Southern Style Tacos (use lettuce leaf not tortilla)

Cooked Veggies
Sweet Potato Fries with Rosemary

Yukon Gold Oven Fries

Grilled Veggie Kabobs

Sample Lunch

Green Salad with Orange Ginger Vinaigrette, Asian Bean Sprout Salad, Rice Paper Wraps, Grilled Veggie Kabobs.

Treat
Phil's Sorbet

At the end of our 21 days we were excited to EAT! We went to a huge buffet at a casino across the street from our house. Phil ordered Prime Rib, soda and all the trimmings. Only a few bites let him know that this was not a good choice, his stomach began to complain and within the next few hours his old friends back pain and diarrhea were back to visit.

My choices to end my detox were bread, pasta and dessert. My body responded very quickly also. My mid back pain returned within about 10 minutes, then my hands began to break out (after being completely clear for most of my detox), and my heels began to hurt (also gone during the detox). The next day we jumped back on our good-food bandwagon and have *continue to be very careful what we eat.*

You will want to add some of the 7 offending foods back into your every day food and some you will eliminate forever, such as chemicals and especially MSG, High Fructose Corn Syrup and artificial sweeteners.

Listen to Your Body
Introduce one food group at a time for 3 days. As you add foods back in, listen to your body, are you having sinus problems? Constipation or diarrhea more aches and pains, headaches, insomnia, emotional or feeling cranky?

Is your skin breaking out, brain fog returning, are you suddenly more anxious? ***These are all signs that the food you are eating is not good for your body.*** Your body is talking, now it is time to listen. Eliminate that particular food again and see if the symptoms clear up.

HOW TO REINTRODUCE FOODS

1. *Stay on the 75% raw 25% cooked and only add one food at a time, for 3 days.*
2. *Keep track of physical changes in a journal.*
3. *After 3 days, stop that food and go back to 75/25 for 3 days to clear your body.*
4. *Add next food.*

After you have tried the foods you want to reintroduce, go to the Detox, ETC plan. Any foods that caused physical symptoms are not good for you and you should be intentional about avoiding them.

<< Knowing what foods affect your body in a negative way is a gift! Follow this procedure to help you stay healthy for life! >>

My "Ah-Ha" moment of how much food affected my body came about 10 days into our detox. Phil & I had a catering job and did not bring food we could eat. I was very hungry and the only thing I could find was a chicken strip (YES! I cheated!). I ate that fried chicken strip and in about 10 minutes my mid back pain returned!

One client came rushing into our office to see the doctor at the end of her detox. She had eaten some salsa at a local Mexican restaurant just minutes before her arrival at our office. Her throat was closing up and hurt like she was getting strep throat. Tomatoes! As an "A" blood type she had avoided tomatoes for 21 days, her body let her know they were not good for her!

Why are we suddenly sensitive? We have put so much junk in our bodies for so many years we can't identify what is causing our "colds", headaches, skin outbreaks, etc. When we remove all those offending foods those symptoms go away.

When we add those offending foods back, we are suddenly aware of what the problem is.

AFTER YOU REINTRODUCE FOODS

OUR LIFE PLAN "DETOX, E.T.C."

Giving your body a break by detoxing is valuable. You feel great, how do you maintain your great and improving health? This is the plan we follow on a regular basis. It is called Detox, Eat, Treat & Celebrate. (Detox, E.T.C.). This plan keeps you on track by clearing your body each week AND allows you to have foods you enjoy on a daily basis and celebration foods once a week. It is a completely livable plan!

One-Day Per Week: (We Do This On Monday)

100% Raw Day – see Days 8-10 of the 28-day detox

Tuesday - Sunday

75/25 Days

PLUS

Choose 1- 3 Per Day Of The Following

Limit to ONE choice if you are on a weight loss track

1 slice Sprouted Grain Bread like Ezekiel or Alvarado Street Bakery bread

1 oz. Raw Cheese or Raw Goat's Cheese

2-3 oz. Organic, Natural Red Meat, Fish, Chicken, Turkey

1-2 Organic eggs

Creamy Salad Dressings such as Ranch

Detox ETC, Menu Ideas

Side Choice

Apple Annie or Garlicky Kale Salad

Broccoli Salad

Asian Citrus Pasta Salad

Sushi Salad

Green Goddess Veggie Sandwich

Protein Choice

Vegetarian Bean Burger

West Coast Fish Tacos

Marvelous Minestrone Soup

Cooked Veggies

Veggie Sauté served with Bean Burger

Veggies in Minestrone Soup

Sample Lunch

Leafy Green Salad with Herb dressing, ½ cup Kale Salad, Green Goddess Veggie Sandwich with 1 Slice Ezekiel Bread, Green Goddess Dressing, Avocado, sliced cucumbers, sliced tomatoes, sliced green onions and 2 inches of baby spinach.

Sample Dinner

Leafy Green Salad with Robb's Italian Balsamic Vinaigrette, Broccoli Salad and Marvelous Minestrone Soup with organic corn muffins.

Detox, Etc. Life Plan Treats

Choose 1-3 per week from any of the Spelt or Dessert Recipes (Only choose zero to one if you are trying to lose weight)

CELEBRATION MEALS

A celebration meal is one meal per week when you eat whatever you like within reason, of course. Celebration meals help you not feel deprived, allow you to live a more normal "food life" with others and keep your metabolism challenged by varying your caloric intake.

The longer you "eat well" the better your choices will be on your celebration days. For instance, if you try a hot dog and it makes you feel sick, next time you might go for a real steak instead of a "tube steak".

<< After your Celebration meal or Celebration day, have a detox day of 100% Raw to clear your body and get right back on track! >>

Celebrate 1 Meal Per Week:

Eat whatever you like, for instance, Pizza, Chicken, mashed potatoes and gravy, enchiladas, etc.

Celebrate 6 days per year:

Eat whatever you like for holidays, vacation days, etc. but also listen to your body. If chocolate gives you migraines, why ruin your celebration? Find a new treat!

Make your celebration choices things you never eat and make most of your celebration food good choices. For instance you might have Pizza and a salad or you might have a steak with wine at dinner or a rich chocolate dessert with your meal.

Alcohol

Coffee

Chocolate

Cheese

Wheat Bread

Refined Sugar

<< *Remember anytime you eat anything with refined sugar or high fructose corn syrup you reduce your immune system function by 60-80% for up to 8 hours. This puts you at risk for catching whatever is going around the office, home or school!* >>

Poisons such as
Non-Sugar Sweeteners, MSG and
Trans Fats are not treats or celebration foods, they are poisons! Always avoid these.

In Their Own Words
"I had an eye exam this week and the doctor reduced my prescription for my glasses! They couldn't explain it but I knew it was a year of drinking carrot juice every day!" JA 40+, F

"When I started my detox I did not like raw vegetables. The Kale Salad was my first favorite. Now I love fresh veggie juice in the morning and my variety of salads every day. I am cured of my bad eating habits. I love my new food!" BM, female, 55 yrs.

CHAPTER 9 FEEDING PEOPLE WHO FEAR CHANGE

Food is a very personal issue for many people, you can tell them what car to buy, where to go on vacation, how to wear their hair but DON'T tell them what to eat! If you want to try to feed your family and friends healthier foods, don't make a big deal about it. Don't look at them fearfully as you announce, "well, I hope you like this, it's really healthy" and hold your breath as you wait for them to take the first bite; they won't even try it out of fear.

The recipes in the following menus are much like prepared foods you would buy but without all the unhealthy additives and preservatives. We take healthy food to our life group dinners twice a month. I used to announce what I brought and what was in it and why it was good for you; no one would touch it until the first brave soul "ventured in". Then someone would say, "hey Celeste, this is really good, what is it?" and suddenly the food would disappear. Now I bring my food in and set it out, I don't even talk about it to my friends, I let it speak for itself, everyone eats it and likes it and those who are interested ask about it.

You wouldn't announce to your family or guests "well, the store was out of Kraft macaroni and cheese so I got the

Kroger brand", would you? Just make the food, act like it is normal and really good (because it is) and they will rave about it. If they don't the first time, keep serving it, they will!

Menus For Special Occasions

Game Day Party

Drinks

Strawberry or Apple Lemonade

Munchies

Better Than Onion Dip

Spicy Hot Dip

Guacamole

Pico de Gallo

Xotchil Organic Corn Chips

Kettle Organic Potato Chips

Fresh Raw Veggies with your dips

Main Dish

Three Bean Chili or Phil's Famous Kitchen Sink Soup

Green Goddess Sandwiches or Organic Corn Muffins

Dessert

Organic Popcorn

Spelt Zucchini Chocolate Chip Muffins

Grandma Davis Chocolate Chip Cookies

Ladies Night Out

Drinks
Mims Cocktail

Starters
Fruit Salad with Lemon Poppy Seed Dip

Veggie Tray

Guacamole

Green Goddess Dip

Main Dish
Butternut Squash Soup

Green Goddess Sandwiches

Refrigerator Apple Muffins or Organic Corn Muffins

Dessert
Gigi's Garden Chocolate Cake with Whip Cream Frosting

Asian Delight

Starters
Bean Sprout Salad on shredded angel hair cabbage

Main Dish
Thai Lettuce Wraps & Asian Salsa

Sweet Orange Stir Fry

Quinoa or Brown Rice

Po-Folk's Dinner for 6
Cheap, quick, healthy and delicious!

Salads

Leaf lettuce tossed in Southwestern Ranch Dressing

Southwestern Slaw

Soup

3 Bean Vegetarian Chili

Bread

Organic Spelt Corn Muffins

Dessert

Baked Apples

Come for Brunch
Holidays, vacations, family events

Drinks

Mims Cocktail

Spicy Tom Cocktail

Salads

Veggie Tray with Real Ranch Dressing Or Green Goddess Dip

Strawberry Pecan Salad

Main Dish – choose one or two items

Spelt Buttermilk Pancakes or Spelt Whole Grain Waffles with fruit compote and warm 100% Maple Syrup.

Turkey Sausage

Oven Roasted Potatoes

Creamy Cashew Gravy or Creamy Turkey Gravy

Mexican Fiesta!
Low Fat Fresh Mexican Favorites

Drinks

Spicy Tom Cocktail

Strawberry Lemonade

Starters

Fresh Pico de Gallo

Fresh Guacamole with sliced Jicama for dipping

Organic Corn Chips

Salads

Southwestern Slaw

Spinach Salad with Warm Garlic Dressing

Main Dish choose one or two

Quinoa Poblano Peppers

Spinach Enchiladas

Chili Relleno Casserole

Southern Style Tacos

Dessert

Nacho Strawberries

Let's Do Lunch
Quick Lunch With Friends And Family

Drinks

Apple Lemonade

Main Dish

Green goddess Sandwich

Phil's Famous Kitchen Sink Soup

Dessert

Raw Peach Cobbler

Favorite Family Menus
Just Make The Food And Let It Speak For Itself

Macaroni & Cheese Please

Drink

Apple Lemonade

Main Dish

Homemade Mac & Cheese

Veggies

A leafy green salad

A cooked veggie

HEALTHIER INGREDIENTS IN YOUR FAVORITE FAMILY RECIPES

Convert your favorite recipes (some of them anyway) to a healthier version by using the following:

Spelt Flour in place of Wheat flour

Spelt, Rice or Quinoa pasta

Quinoa or brown rice in place of couscous or pasta

Grape seed Oil or Unrefined Extra Virgin Coconut Oil for cooking

Almond, Coconut or Hemp milk in place of cow's milk

Celtic Sea Salt in place of table Celtic Sea Salt

Raw Honey or Coconut sugar in place of white or brown sugar

Cage Free Eggs or Enr-G Egg replacement

Olive oil for uncooked recipes like salad dressings or put on food after it is cooked

Rumford's Aluminum Free Baking Powder & Bob's Red Mill Aluminum Free Baking Soda

Organic soups, sauces and canned goods

Raw cheeses, sparingly

Grass Fed Beef

Free Range Chickens

Wild Caught Fish

It's Not Hard, It's Just Different!

The most difficult part of change is the process involved in change, the fact that you must THINK about doing things you had previously done without thinking. For instance, currently, if you are hungry, you do what you have always done, look for convenient foods you have always eaten.

As you begin to eat for health and nutrition, you have to THINK about the food you are going to eat, where you are going to get it or how you are going to make it. You may have to learn some new ways of creating food; this is the process that can be difficult part for you. For your family the difficulty of change is tradition and texture; not so much taste, taste is not intrinsic it is learned.

<< *Raw foods are easy. Choose the foods you like, add a dressing flavor you like and you have a meal!* >>

For instance, your family may be used to going through the drive through every time they have a ball game, which is tradition. They love the taste of fast food because it is familiar to them and because of the thousands of chemicals in fast food that make you think it tastes good. If you suddenly stop going out for fast food after a game you are changing tradition. To make the change more pleasant, start a new tradition, for instance, have a picnic at the field after the game with food you bring, invite another family to join you. You could also have food ready at home after the game and sit around the table and talk about the great time you had. If you create new traditions with healthier versions of the food they love, it won't be as difficult. Your family will learn to love the new foods you make if you do it slowly and lovingly, not like a drill sergeant.

Convert the family slowly and remember children do not have the knowledge and wisdom to choose their own food. You are the adult; you are the one with the knowledge and wisdom. Here are some things to remember about changing the family food.

Do not ask anyone in your family to eat anything you will not eat yourself; it won't work.

Do not bribe, threaten or cajole, do not even let them know you are changing, just do it. Currently you don't inform them when you buy a different brand of Baking Powder or different tomato sauces so don't make a big deal about these changes.

Start by mixing small amounts of the thing you want to change, gradually increase the good ingredient. Example: Start using goat, almond, coconut or hemp milk by adding a little of the alternative milk to your regular milk, slowly increase the alternative milk and decrease cow's milk. Flour; slowly start replacing white regular flour with white spelt flour. Once you make that switch, start replacing the white spelt flour with small amounts of whole grain spelt.

Try one new thing; keep offering it until they accept it. Taste is not intrinsic, it is acquired. They currently have a taste for the foods they have always eaten. Eventually they will have a taste for the new foods. It takes 10-15 times before a child will accept a new food.

In her book Unhealthy Truth, Robyn O'Brien tells of switching her four children to healthy yogurt. She learned about the dangers of food dyes and decided, "no more blue yogurt"! So she bought the healthier plain yogurt with no dyes, sugar or high fructose corn syrup. She told the kids they could make up their own yogurt creations with sprinkles (the kind you put on cookies). She let them go to town with the sprinkles, she just wanted them to get used to the white yogurt. After a few days of white yogurt with sprinkles, suddenly one day they just "ran out of sprinkles". "Oh no", she told her children, "I guess we'll just have to try it with fruit today". From then on they ate white yogurt with fresh fruit and forgot about the sprinkles! No battles!

When introducing new foods, require your children to try one spoonful of the new food each time you make it.

Do not become a short order cook. If the food you are making is tasty and healthy, do not apologize or offer anything else. Eat this or wait until the next meal to eat what I prepare then. There are no medical records of children starving to death because they refused to eat. When they get hungry, they will eat what you allow or provide, it's up to you. Be strong, it is for their ultimate good.

As your family accepts one new thing, for instance salads, then begin to offer them several times a week. When you have completely switched to spelt flour, don't go back to wheat flour, and only use spelt. As your family fully accepts an item, keep it and begin something new.

My Spouse Doesn't Share My Views On Food
Unfortunately, this is a common problem but it can be navigated successfully. We all have the foods we are used to and for many adults and some children, giving up our favorite foods are a complex and sometimes emotional issue. Again, start with yourself, when your spouse, children and friends see the great changes in your body and your health, they will want to try your food, don't push, model.

If your spouse refuses to allow you to change the family food, just work on your own meals, eating more fresh veggies and fruits. You can also change things they won't notice, like using some organic Ingredients. Eventually, if the changes you make affect you in a positive way, those changes will also impact your family and they will be more open to change themselves.

Prayer is always a valuable tool for any situation. Ask God to speak to your spouse and children about accepting healthy foods. Ask Him to give you ideas of new, healthier foods your family will accept and enjoy.

Many times women will "drag" their husbands to meet with us to learn about healthy eating. Usually these women want to make changes themselves and are concerned about their husband's health as well. A wife will get me to the side and say "I doubt he will do this but I'm doing it whether he does or not." At the end of our meeting, after learning the truth about food, the husband will look at the wife and say something like "I don't know about you but I'm definitely doing this healthy eating stuff".

Spouses and children generally respond well to truth. Rather than sharing facts you are learning, just do it yourself. Your family and friends will begin to see the positive changes in your own life. Your personal testimony will allow them to receive truth and change much more quickly than badgering them or manipulating them.

SIMPLE EVERYDAY CHANGES

White Spelt flour instead of white flour

Rice or spelt angel hair spaghetti instead of traditional angel hair spaghetti

Rice, spelt or quinoa pasta shells, macaroni, etc. instead of traditional pasta

Enjoy Life brand chocolate chips (or an organic brand) instead of your usual brand

Raw cheese instead of pasteurized cheese

Organic butter instead of margarine or regular butter

Organic dairy products

Better Than Bouillon brand instead of regular Bouillon

Celtic Sea Salt instead of regular Sea Salt

Organic corn products and snack items

Homemade yogurt or **Erivan Yogurt** *made with unpasteurized milk, instead of regular and add fresh fruit and raw local honey to sweeten.*

Natural nitrate free hot dogs and deli meats

Natural, grass feed beef, free-range chicken and wild caught fish

Cage free, natural eggs

Sucanat or organic sugar instead of regular sugar and brown sugar

Local Raw honey or Coconut sugar instead of refined sugar

In Their Own Words

"My kids LOVE the Homemade Macaroni & Cheese, the Spelt Chocolate Chip Zucchini Muffins and the Broccoli Salad, YAY!"

WONDERFULLY WELL

A COLLECTION OF WHOLE FOOD RECIPES AND MENUS FROM THE WELLNESS WORKSHOP

Psalm 139:14

I will praise You for I am fearfully and wonderfully made.

Marvelous are Your works and that my soul knows very well.

NUTRITION KEY FOR RECIPES

These symbols are next to each recipe name.

GF   Gluten Free

DF   Dairy Free

SF   Sugar Free

NSO   Natural Sugar Only

HF   High Fiber

HP   High Protein

LF   Low Fat

BF   Beneficial Fats

NV (all recipes are vegan unless marked NV

Check the Index for:

Cleanse/Detox Recipes

CHAPTER 10 FRESH JUICES AND SMOOTHIES GF, DF, NSO

Only use Organic fruits and veggies for your juice to avoid over exposure to pesticides and chemicals and get maximum nutritional value. Remove peels of non-organics.

DAILY JUICES

Drink a minimum of 16 ounces of fresh vegetable juice a day.

Daily Antioxidant Juice

Phil Davis (makes approximately 16 ounces)
This is our daily juice; we drink approximately 16 ounces per day.

Ingredients

    1 pound juicing carrots (4-8), peeled if desired
    1 gala or honey crisp apple (you can use whatever you like)
    ¼ lemon, peeled

Instructions

Wash all, cut apple in chunks to go through juicer, peel lemon, put through juicer, stir and drink within 20 minutes. Juice made in a Champion or Omega can be kept sealed in a glass jar in the refrigerator for up to 24 hours. Green Star, can be kept up to 72 hours.

For added cleansing, add one or more of these to the Daily Antioxidant juice:
    ¼ beet
    2 stalks celery
    2 stalks Kale

Make it Green

Alternate leafy greens with carrots or apples to avoid jamming the juicer.
    Replace carrots with 1 head of romaine or celery
    Add some Kale (5-6 stalks)
    1 to 2 inches fresh Ginger if you like it

There are many juice books available; we use **Fresh Vegetable and Fruit Juices** by Norman Walker as it has proven combinations to help the body heal from many health related conditions.

8 veggies Juice

Celeste Davis
Ah...summer is the best time for this refreshing, hydrating juice with fresh from the garden tomatoes.

Run clean veggies through juicer
    3 organic fresh tomatoes
    1 clove garlic
    1 banana pepper
    ¼ green pepper
    2 celery stalks
    1 small cucumber
    1-2 green onions
    ¼ lemon (peeled)

Adjust Ingredients to taste.

Spicy Tom

Celeste Davis (serves 2)
A delicious non-alcoholic bloody Mary.

Run clean veggies through juicer

    4 organic tomatoes
    ½ organic cucumber
    ¼ green pepper or jalapeno
    1 garlic clove
    2 celery stalks
    Dash Tabasco sauce or sprinkle with ground cayenne, just a touch!

Serve over ice

Thanksgiving Cocktail

Phil Davis Makes about 1 ½ quarts
Your family and guests will rave about this juice.

Run clean fruits through juicer

    8 new crop apples like Honey Crisp or Gala
    2 bags raw fresh cranberries
    4 lbs. purple grapes
    ¼ to 1 lemon (to taste)

Serve over ice

Make it sparkling by adding Gerolstiener sparkling filtered water to taste.

Apple Lemonade

Phil Davis (serves 2-3)
Another family favorite, one glass is plenty of this very cleansing juice.

Run clean fruits through juicer

5 organic apples (we like Pink Lady)
1 organic lemon

Serve over ice or combine with Gerolstiener Mineral Water to taste for a carbonated drink.

Strawberry Lemonade

Phil Davis (serves 4-6)
This is a sweet refreshing summer time treat. Keep it on hand to replace sodas. Add a tea bag for a twist.

Ingredients

1-cup fresh lemon juice (about 3 lemons) (peel all but about ¼ of 1 lemon)
1-pint strawberries
¼ to ½ cup raw local honey (adjust to taste)
4 cups water to desired taste
(to make sparkling, substitute 2 cups of filtered water with Gerolstiener sparkling filtered water. Pour Gerolstiener slowly as it will bubble up, make sure you have a large pitcher.)

Instructions

Juice lemons in your juicer.
Blend strawberries and raw agave in a magic bullet.
Mix lemon juice, filtered water and strawberry/agave mixture, adjust to taste. Stir Well.

Dehydration is a serious potential danger, especially with vomiting and diarrhea. Many people use Gatorade to prevent dehydration. This drink does have electrolytes, however, it is also high in sugar, which suppresses the immune system. Try one of these juices instead, many of our clients rave about them.

Cold & Flu Juice

Make the basic juice and add Ingredients according to your symptoms.

Ingredients

> 2 lemons
> 1 apple
> 1 pear
> 2 slices of fresh pineapple
> 1-cup hot filtered water
> 1 Tablespoon RAW honey (do not give honey to children under 2 yrs. of age)

Instructions

Run fruit through juicer, mix hot water honey, stir in juice. Add one or more of the following to the basic juice.

For upset stomach add:

> 1 knob fresh, peeled ginger (about 1 inch), (soothing to stomach)
> Run through juicer with fruit
> 1/8 teaspoon ground nutmeg or cardamom (flavor, soothing to stomach)
> ¼ teaspoon ground anise (gas, cramping)

For sinus and congestion add:

> ¼ teaspoon cinnamon OR 1 clove garlic (to fight infection)
> ¼ tsp ground anise seed (for cough)
> Sprinkle cayenne pepper (to boost immune system &clear sinus)

Many of our clients are sold on these healing and cleansing juices when a cold strikes. Please consult with a licensed medical professional for all matters pertaining to your health. It is excellent for children and adults (note honey warning for children under age 2). Add the spices you choose a little at a time until you like the flavor.
** All children should be seen by a health care professional to exclude serious causes of fever such as meningitis.

Ginger is great for nausea. Herbal ginger tea is comforting and calms the stomach. Get a natural ginger ale and avoid ginger ale with high fructose corn syrup and artificial ginger.

To boost immunity make the antioxidant juice but add a handful of parsley, 1 clove of garlic and 3 stalks of celery.

Wallyade - Alkalizing Sports Drink

Phil Davis (makes approx ½ gallon)
The first ingredient of the popular "ade" sports drink is high fructose corn syrup. Need we say more?

This juice is full of natural electrolytes your body can store. It can virtually eliminate the aches and pains after workouts. Drink 8 oz. immediately after workout. Wait 20 minutes; eat beans or nuts for protein.

Ingredients
> ½ small watermelon with rind and seeds, wash well
> 1 mango, peeled
> 1 lime, peeled
> 1 lemon peeled
> 1 to 5 oranges, peeled (according to your taste)
> 1-cup fresh pineapple

Wallyade Juice Instructions
Run all through juicer, put into 8 oz. glass jars, filled to top, seal and store in fridge. If you are going to freeze leave 1 inch at top of jar for expansion of juice.

<< We use Wallyade juice after our work out and never have muscle aches; it is also good for colds >>

SMOOTHIES

Barney Smoothie

Celeste Davis (serves one)
You don't have to spend big bucks on a protein shake. This is a delicious, nutritious, smoothie everyone will love. No one will know there is raw spinach in it!

Ingredients
1 frozen banana
½ cup frozen blueberries
1 handful raw baby spinach
2 drops liquid Stevia will make it really sweet
Coconut, Hemp or Almond milk
1 teaspoon Flaxseed oil

Instructions
Cut banana in chunks, place all Ingredients except oil in magic bullet or blender, blend on high until smooth, and add oil, pulse to blend, drink immediately.

For a protein shake add to your smoothie:
2 Tablespoons ground flaxseed (grind first in magic bullet or coffee grinder)
3 Tablespoons ground hemp seeds (grind first in magic bullet or coffee grinder)

Puree all in blender or magic bullet. Add alternative milk to desired consistency.

Flaxseed Smoothie

Celeste Davis (serves one)
Flaxseeds are known to be beneficial for cancer prevention. Studies have shown that breast cancer survivors who eat 3 Tablespoons of

177

flaxseeds per day have better cancer protection with fewer side effects than those who take Tamoxifen. Flaxseeds are beneficial for anyone, whether or not they have had cancer. DO NOT BUY FLAX MEAL as it is just a by-product of flaxseed oil and does not have the benefit of the whole flaxseed.

Ingredients

    2-3 Tablespoons whole organic flaxseeds
    ½ cup filtered water

Instructions

Grind flaxseeds DRY in magic bullet or coffee grinder to a fine powder. Add filtered water and blend well. Set aside for 10 minutes to gel. Mixture will become thick. Drink after 10 minutes.

Maca Shooter

Celeste Davis (serves one)
Maca is a root vegetable from Peru known to rebuild weak organs. It is especially helpful for the adrenal glands to increase stamina and male and female reproductive systems. It can help with infertility and low libido in both men and women. Use for 3 months, and then discontinue.

Ingredients

    1 teaspoon Maca powder (we like Nativas brand)
    ¼ cup filtered water

Instructions

Blend Maca and filtered water in magic bullet or blender until well blended. Drink immediately. We shoot it, because it tastes terrible!

All Salad Dressings in this book are Gluten Free

CHAPTER 11   DRESSING, DIPS AND MARINADES, GF

Salad dressings can give you more calories and hidden toxins than any other thing you put in your mouth! Bottled dressings also tend to be full of preservatives, high fructose corn syrup, EDTA, MSG and other extremely harmful chemicals. Make your own, it's quick, easy and delicious and less expensive!

Avoid commercial salad dressings are made with genetically modified oils: Corn Oil, Canola Oil, Cottonseed Oil, and Soybean Oil. The corn, rapeseed, cottonseed and soybeans are genetically modified with the weed killer roundup...need we say more? They store as FAT in your body because they are toxins.

Flaxseed oil is the only oil that is used immediately by the body and does not store as fat, use it as often as possible in place of any oils in salad dressings. It is also great for your skin, brain, hair and nails! Don't cook with it.

Use Olive Oil and Grape seed oil in any salad dressing.

How much dressing should you use? The best way to moderate salad dressing is to pour 1-2 Tablespoons over your salad and toss it, like they do in the restaurant.

CREAMY DRESSINGS

Quick Fresh Guacamole GF, SF, BF
Celeste Davis (makes ½ cup)
Ingredients
  1 Large avocado
  2 Tablespoons Pico de Gallo
  1 clove garlic
  Juice of ½ a fresh lime
  Celtic Sea Salt

Instructions
Mince garlic, Cut avocado in chunks and mash with a fork or run through a food processor, stir in Pico de Gallo, garlic and lime. Salt to taste.

About Avocados
Avocado is a GREAT fat choice. 1/8 of an avocado is equal to one of your daily fat servings. Studies have shown avocado to significantly decrease LDL cholesterol and increase HDL cholesterol. It is also great for skin and hair. Avocado has the highest enzyme count of any fresh fruit.

CHOOSING AN AVOCADO
To open an avocado, cut in half, remove seed and use a spoon to remove fruit, for chunks carefully run a knife through the avocado without piercing the skin, cut both ways, like you would cut a pan of brownies. Spoon out and you will have chunks. Leave seed in half an avocado and save in crisper in fridge, remove browned top before serving.

Real Ranch Dressing GF, SF , NV

Celeste Davis (makes 2 cups)
Better taste than any bottle you will ever open! No harmful preservatives and MSG AND your family will love it. Make ahead; flavor is better the next day, can be kept for 3-5 days.

Ingredients

> 1-cup goat or Greek yogurt
> 1-cup Veganaise (made with Grape seed oil)
> 1 teaspoon Celtic Sea Salt
> 1-teaspoon garlic granules
> 1-teaspoon onion granules
> 1 teaspoon dried parsley flakes
> 1 teaspoon dried thyme

Instructions

Blend all in magic bullet, blender or food processor.

Refrigerate in sealed glass jar for up to 7 days. Use as dip, dressing or sandwich spread.

Variations

Blue Cheese – crumble blue cheese or feta into dressing

Dill – add 1-teaspoon dry dill or 1 Tablespoon fresh dill

Basil Dill – add 1 Tablespoon fresh dill and 1 Tablespoon fresh basil

Green Goddess – add 3 green onions tops and all, 1- 3 garlic cloves, 1-2 Tablespoons fresh dill and 3-4 fresh basil leaves and 1 teaspoon organic Dijon mustard. Blend in food processor, blender or magic bullet. This is always a crowd pleaser.

Creamy Southwest Ranch Dressing GF, DF, SF

Celeste Davis
This is delicious on fine sliced, angel hair cabbage or chopped veggies served with West Coast Fish Tacos or 3 Bean Chili.

Ingredients
    1 Roma tomato, chopped
    1 jalapeno pepper, seeded & chopped
    1 clove garlic, chopped or ½ teaspoon minced garlic
    2-4 Tablespoons Grape seed Veganaise

Instructions
Put all in blender or magic bullet and blend well. For chopped veggie salad, put on a variety of chopped veggies, serve over greens.

Creamy Lime Dressing GF, SF

Celeste Davis (makes 1 cup)
Excellent on Jicama salad and thinly sliced cabbage.

Ingredients
    1-cup plain goat or Greek yogurt or Erivan's Yogurt
    1 Tablespoon chopped fresh cilantro
    1 Tablespoon   thinly sliced fresh green onion
    2 teaspoons to 1 Tablespoon fresh limejuice
    Celtic Sea Salt to taste

Instructions
Mix all Ingredients well, store in sealed glass jar in refrigerator for up to 5 days. Use for salads, dips, and Jicama Salad.

Asian Salad Dressing GF, DF, BF

Celeste Davis (makes ¾ cup)
This is great on cabbage or broccoli slaw as well as veggie or green salads. Serve with a stir-fry or as a dipping sauce for rice paper wraps.

Ingredients

¼ cup rice vinegar (can use red wine vinegar)
1 Tablespoon Tamari or Braggs Amino Acids (no MSG soy sauce-use gluten free soy sauce if needed)
½ cup Grape seed or EV Olive Oil
2-3 drops toasted sesame oil (optional)
2 Tablespoons toasted sesame seeds

Instructions

Wisk all together, store in refrigerator for 3-5 days

Nutty Asian Sweet & Hot Dressing GF, DF, NSO, BF

Celeste Davis (makes about 2 cups)
Excellent on the Asian Cabbage salad.

Ingredients

3 Tablespoons Tahini, crunchy almond butter or cashew butter (or combination)
2 Tablespoons Braggs Amino Acids
1 Tablespoon Asian hot red pepper oil
1-teaspoon cayenne
1-teaspoon raw honey
1 teaspoon to 1 Tablespoon toasted sesame oil (add slowly to taste)
2 Tablespoons olive or grape seed oil
1 Tablespoon minced fresh ginger

Nutty Asian Sweet & Hot Dressing continued

1 Tablespoon minced green onion
1 Tablespoon Organic white grape or apple juice
1-teaspoon hot mustard (optional)
½ teaspoon Celtic Sea Salt
1 Tablespoon Better than Bouillon Vegetarian
Vegetable base
1 ½ cups water

Instructions

Put all Ingredients in magic bullet, mix well. Store in a glass jar in refrigerator for up to one week. Excellent on angel hair cabbage or bean sprout salad, or as a dipping sauce for rice paper wraps.

Dijon Mustard Vinaigrette GF, DF, SF, BF

Celeste Davis (makes about 1 cup)
This is a Davis household staple.

Ingredients

1/4 cup red wine vinegar or Braggs Raw Apple Cider Vinegar
3 Tablespoons extra virgin expeller pressed olive oil
1-3 small garlic cloves, minced
2 teaspoons Dijon mustard
1/4 Tablespoon minced fresh oregano (or 1 teaspoon dried)
1/4 teaspoon Celtic Sea Salt
1/4 teaspoon freshly ground pepper

Instructions

Mince garlic in magic bullet or by hand. Add other Ingredients, slowly whisk in olive oil.

Red Wine Vinaigrette Dressing GF, DF, SF, BF

Celeste Davis (makes about 1 cup)
A low fat version, we keep this handy for our daily 4 handfuls of leafy greens.

Ingredients

    8 Tablespoons filtered water
    4 Tablespoons Red Wine Vinegar
    2 Tablespoons Rice Vinegar
    4 Tablespoons Grape seed or Extra Virgin Olive Oil
    (Expeller pressed)
    2 teaspoons Dijon mustard
    ¼ teaspoon Red pepper flakes
    ½ teaspoon Italian seasoning
    Pinch of Celtic Sea Salt

    For Asian flavor eliminate Celtic Sea Salt and add:
    *Splash (1/4 – ½ teaspoon) toasted Sesame Oil
    (optional)
    *½ - 1 Tablespoon Braggs Amino Acids (optional)

Instructions

Combine all Ingredients and mix well. With a wire whisk, whisk in oil until well blended. This can also be made in magic bullet by combining all and blending in bullet.

Robb's Italian Balsamic Dressing GF, DF, NSO, BF

Robb Davis (makes about 1 cup)
Playing with food is a Davis family hobby; this is from our son, Robb.

Ingredients

6 Tablespoons cold pressed extra virgin olive oil
¼ - ½ cup organic balsamic vinegar (we like the light balsamic infused with pomegranate)
2 pinches Celtic Sea Salt
1 Tablespoon minced garlic
1 Tablespoon minced red onion
1 Tablespoon minced sweet yellow onion
1 Tablespoon minced sun dried tomatoes

Instructions

The best way to mince veggies is to put in a food processor or magic bullet. Whisk all Ingredients together. Serve over crisp romaine and fresh veggies. Toss well. Store in sealed glass jar, in refrigerator for up to 1 week in fridge.

Lime Dressing GF, DF, NSO, BF

Celeste Davis (makes about ¼ cup)
This is one of my everyday favorites, especially on cabbage.

Ingredients

2-3 Tablespoons fresh limejuice (1-2 limes)
2 Tablespoons flax seed oil
1/8 teaspoon ground red chili pepper
2 Tablespoons raw local honey
2 Tablespoons red onion, minced

Instructions

Blend well in magic bullet. Keep in fridge 3-5 days.

Herb Dressing GF, DF, NSO, BF

Celeste Davis (makes about 1 cup)
This is a tangy sweet dressing. You can pack it with more fresh herbs for extra zing!

Ingredients

1/3-cup fresh squeezed lemon juice
1-3 Tablespoons raw local honey (adjust to taste)
1-3 garlic cloves (to taste)
1 teaspoon dry basil or 1 Tablespoon fresh basil
1/3 cup distilled filtered water
¼ teaspoon Celtic Sea Salt
1 Tablespoon red or yellow onion (if onion is strong use less)
1 Tablespoon oregano
1 teaspoon crushed red pepper flakes (optional)

Instructions

Put onion and garlic in magic bullet or food processor and mince fine, combine with liquids. Set aside on counter for several hours before serving so flavors can blend.

Roasted Garlic Dressing GF, DF, SF, BF

Celeste Davis
A Whole Foods class favorite, wonderful on salads, roasted veggies or grilled fish or chicken.

Ingredients

2 Tablespoons Braggs Raw Apple Cider Vinegar
3 Tablespoons Grape seed oil
2 Tablespoons grated Raw Parmesan Cheese or Parmesan Reggiano (raw Parmesan)
1 full head of garlic, roasted

Instructions

Squeeze the soft, cooked garlic into a food processor or blender; add other Ingredients, blend until smooth. You can also add fresh basil or dill to this recipe.

How to Roast Garlic   GF, DF, SF

You can do one head of garlic at a time or many heads of garlic at once.

Take the whole head of garlic and cut about ¼ to ½ inch off the pointy top (the bottom has a root on it), you will be able to see the tops of each clove of garlic.

Line the cup of a muffin pan with enough foil to wrap the garlic and place cut head of garlic inside foil, cut side up.

Drizzle a couple of teaspoons of Grape seed oil over each garlic head.

Close the foil over the garlic head. Bake at 400°degrees F for 30-35 minutes, or until the cloves feel soft when pressed. Roast several garlic heads at once and use one for garlic butter or to mix with your steamed veggies....yummy!

Roasted Red Pepper Vinaigrette GF, DF, NSO, BF

Celeste Davis (makes about 1 cup)
It's not as hard as it sounds!

Ingredients
> 2 medium red bell peppers
> 2 Tablespoons sherry vinegar
> 1 garlic clove, crushed
> 1/3 cup filtered water
> 1 Tablespoon olive oil
> Celtic Sea Salt
> Fresh ground white or red pepper (not black)

Instructions
Roast the red pepper, see directions following this recipe.

Make the dressing: In a food processor combine peppers, vinegar, 1/3 cup filtered water, garlic, Celtic Sea Salt and pepper and blend until very smooth. With machine still running, drizzle in olive oil. Season to taste with Celtic Sea Salt and pepper.

How To Roast Red Pepper GF, DF, SF

Set oven to Broil. You can do one pepper at a time or many at once and freeze the ones you don't use.

Brush clean peppers on all sides with a little Grape seed oil (about 1 tsp per pepper)

Place peppers on a baking sheet and put into oven on top rack.

Watch peppers, every few minutes, as they will brown quickly. As one side gets dark spots, turn over with tongs until the whole pepper has large dark spots, you don't want to burn all the way through, just the skin is dark.

Remove from oven and place in a glass dish with a lid for 15 minutes. Peppers will cool and skin will remove easily.

After 15 minutes, grabbing stem, pull stem and seeds out of pepper and discard the stem and seeds. Using the blunt side of a knife, scrape outside to remove skin or peel it off like old nail polish.

Cut pepper in half and use blunt side of knife to scrape out remaining seeds or membrane that is sticking up.

Roast several heads of garlic and red peppers at once, store separately in sealed glass container in refrigerator for 3 days or in zip loc Baggies in freezer for 1 month, use in recipes as needed.

Cherry Balsamic Vinaigrette GF, DF, NSO, BF

Celeste Davis (makes about 2 cups)
This is a cooking class favorite.

Ingredients
1 cup frozen dark sweet cherries, thawed and drained
3 Tablespoons Grape seed oil
½ cup pomegranate infused light balsamic vinegar
1 Tablespoon chopped shallots or green onions
1 Tablespoon apple cider vinegar
Celtic Sea Salt & pepper to taste

Instructions
Combine all in magic bullet or blender and blend well, add a sprig of fresh rosemary for extra flavor, remove rosemary before serving. Store in sealed glass jar in the refrigerator for up to one week.

Serve with a salad of spring mixed greens, red onion, dried cherries, feta and sweet & spicy pecans.

Cherry Salsa GF, DF, NSO, BF

Celeste Davis (makes about 4 cups)
A great addition to salads or as a dip.

Ingredients
4 or 5 medium-size tomatoes (ripe but firm)
1 pint pitted, sweet Bing cherries* (or other sweet fruit-peach, mango, pineapple are good)
½ bunch cilantro (less if you are not a cilantro fan)
4 green onions or ¼ cup chopped red onion
1 large clove garlic
**make it spicy with a half fresh jalapeno seeded and minced

Cherry Salsa Instructions continued

Chop tomatoes and peppers into small chunks. Use S-blade on food processor if you have one, Chop Cilantro, and then add peppers, onions and then tomatoes. Pulse a few times after each addition. Add tomatoes last and pulse to fine chop.

Serve immediately, or cover and refrigerate for later. Will keep about 3 days Use like any salsa on salads or as a veggie dip.

Cranberry Vinaigrette GF, DF, NSO, BF

Makes 2 ½ cups
Inspired by a recipe from the November 2000 issue of Vegetarian Times. This is a wonderful fall and winter salad dressing, best with raw cranberries. Use on Spinach Poppy Seed salad instead of Poppy Seed dressing or on the Fall Salad, you'll find all the raw salads in Chapter 12.
To soften dried cranberries, cover with boiling filtered water and let stand for 15 minutes. Drain before using.

Ingredients

1 ½ cup fresh or reconstituted dried cranberries (Eden's organics are sugar free & unsulphured)
1-cup apple cider (not vinegar)
¼ - 1/3 cup raw local honey
1/3-cup olive oil or Grape seed oil
1 Tablespoon Dijon mustard
1 ½ teaspoon Braggs Raw Apple Cider Vinegar
1 teaspoon Celtic Sea Salt
1/8 teaspoon dried red peppers

Instructions

Combine all in blender or magic bullet, blend until smooth. Store in sealed glass jar in refrigerator for 3-5 days

Fruit Compote GF, DF, NSO

Celeste Davis (serves one person)
Use on waffles, pancakes, and ice cream! Amount of fruit used will depend on how many servings you need, allow approximately ¼ cup compote per serving.

Ingredients
- ¼ cup Fresh or frozen berries (any kind but don't mix blueberries and other berries).
- 1-2 Tablespoons (to taste) raw local honey

Instructions
In food processor, using S blade, pulse chop berries (don't puree). Stir in raw agave nectar (to taste). Warm on stove until syrup-like, don't boil. Easy Way! Put in a small crock-pot; turn on 30 min before serving (turn on low, watch)

** Keep it low fat by adding 1 Tablespoon of butter just before serving, that way people don't have to put butter on their pancakes or waffles but will have a nice buttery flavor.

Orange Ginger Vinaigrette GF, DF, SF, BF

Celeste Davis (makes about ½ cup)
This is the signature dressing for my Sushi Salad; however it can be used for stir-fry, marinated veggie salads or pasta salads as well. Serve it with your 2 handfuls of greens, shredded Jicama, Clementine's and almonds.

Ingredients
- 1/4-cup fresh orange juice
- 1/4 cup Grape seed oil or unrefined coconut oil
- 1 Tablespoon grated fresh ginger (preferred) or ¼ teaspoon ground ginger
- 1-teaspoon fresh grated garlic
- 1-teaspoon brown mustard

Orange Ginger Vinaigrette Continued
>1 teaspoon Braggs Amino Acids
>1/4 teaspoon freshly ground white or red pepper

Instructions
Mix Ingredients in magic bullet.

Note: If you use coconut oil it will solidify if your other Ingredients are cold. Set coconut oil jar warm water for a few minutes to liquefy oil. For best results all ingredients should be room temperature.

Refrigerate and use within 3 days. Excellent!

Berry Lemon Poppy Seed Dressing GF, NSO, BF

Celeste Davis (makes about 2 ½ cups)
Use this as a dressing for fruit salad or spinach salad.

Ingredients
>1/3-cup fresh lemon juice
>1 cup pureed fresh strawberries (or any berry)
>1 teaspoon Dijon mustard
>1 teaspoon Celtic Sea Salt
>¼ cup (start with less) raw local honey
>3/4 cup extra virgin olive oil or Grape seed Oil
>2 Tablespoons Poppy Seeds

Instructions
Put all Ingredients in magic bullet or blender and blend well. Store in sealed glass jar in refrigerator for up to one week. Serve with Spinach Strawberry Salad.

Sweet and Sour Dressing GF, DF, NSO, BF

Celeste Davis
This is a great dressing for the 3-Minute Salad

Ingredients

¼ cup Braggs Raw Apple Cider Vinegar
3 Tablespoons raw local honey
1 Tablespoon minced garlic
1 Tablespoon minced onion
4 Tablespoons flaxseed or Grape seed oil
1 teaspoon red chili pepper flakes

Instructions

Blend in magic bullet and pour over a mixture of your favorite chopped veggies and marinate for at least 1 hour.

VEGGIE DIPS & MARINADES

Many packaged dips and marinades are full of preservatives, high fructose corn syrup, EDTA, MSG and other extremely harmful chemicals. Make your own, it's quick, easy and delicious.

Serve these delicious dips with fresh raw veggies, non-GMO corn chips, or rice crackers.

AUNT CELESTE'S PARTY DIPS

Basic Party Dip GF, NSO, NV

Celeste Davis
This is the basic dip for "Better-Than Onion, Spicy Hot and Lemon Poppy Seed Dips. Make up your own favorites by adding fresh herbs and flavors.

Basic Party Dip Ingredients
 1 ½ cups Grape seed Veganaise
 1 6 oz. carton plain Greek or goat yogurt

Instructions
Mix well, allow flavors to blend overnight for best flavor. Store in sealed glass jar in refrigerator for up to one week.

Tami's Homemade Yogurt GF

Contributed by Tami Hollis (makes 2 quarts)
Quick, Simple, Healthy and Delicious!
Ingredients
 ½ gallon organic whole milk
 ¼ cup plain yogurt

Tips
- Erivan Yogurt at Health food markets is best, Oikos Greek Yogurt would be second best
- Non-homogenized milk is better also!
- Only use whole milk!
- To sweeten, add honey after it is made. Make your own "fruit yogurt" with blended fresh fruit and honey!

Instructions
Pour a half-gallon of organic milk into a large glass jar (preferably a wide-mouth). Stir in ¼ c plain yogurt – the best you can find in the grocery. Place it in the oven. Turn the oven on set at 200 degrees. When oven reaches 200, turn the oven off and leave the door closed for 24 hours. Voila", beautiful yogurt. Save ¼ cup yogurt from each batch to make a new batch. Store in glass jar in refrigerator.

Health Tip! Most commercial yogurts contain a bacteria, s.thermophilus, which is known to stimulate autoimmune disease. Check the ingredients of your yogurt.

Creamy Onion Dip GF

Tastes better than packaged "French Onion Dip"

Ingredients

  1 recipe basic dip
  ¾ teaspoon garlic powder (not Celtic Sea Salt)
  1 Tablespoon Better Than Bouillon
  1 Tablespoon onion powder
  1 Tablespoon dried parsley
  6 Tablespoons dried onion flakes (also called minced onion)

Instructions

Mix basic dip recipe; add all Ingredients, mix well, stir in onion flakes. Refrigerate, best if it sits for 24 hours for flavors to blend and onion to soften.

Spicy Hot Dip GF

Ingredients

  1 recipe basic dip
  1 Tablespoon Better than Bouillon
  ½ teaspoon crushed red pepper flakes
  1/3 to ½ teaspoon white pepper or cayenne (use sparingly)

Instructions

Mix well, refrigerate until serving. Store in sealed glass jar for up to one week. Serve as veggie, chip dip or salad dressing. Spicy Hot Dip is also good as topping for veggie burgers.

Lemon Poppy Seed Dip GF

Sweet dip for fruits and veggies, fruit salads, even chips

Ingredients

  1 recipe basic dip
  2-6 Tablespoons raw agave nectar or raw honey
  3 Tablespoons lemon juice
  Zest of one lemon
  2 Tablespoons Poppy Seeds

Instructions

Mix well, refrigerate until serving. Store in sealed glass jar in refrigerator for up to one week.

Green Goddess Dip & Sandwich Spread GF, DF, SF, BF

Celeste Davis (makes 1 ½ cups)
This is my signature dressing, it is to die for! This recipe was invented on the spot at a Whole Foods cooking class when we had more people than food. It was a huge hit. You and your family will love it on vegetarian sandwiches, veggie burgers and as a dip for relish trays.

Ingredients

  1-cup grape seed Veganaise
  3 green onions cut off root and chop in small pieces
  3 large garlic cloves
  5 leaves fresh basil or 1 teaspoon dried (fresh is best)
  2 inches fresh dill, stem removed or 1 teaspoon dried (again, fresh is best)
  2 Tablespoons lemon juice or Braggs Raw Apple Cider Vinegar

Instructions

Put all in a magic bullet or food processor in the above order and blend until pureed. May need to open jar and move food around or add a little more lemon juice or vinegar to get it moving. Store in sealed glass jar in refrigerator for up to one week.

Pico de Gallo GF, DF, NSO, BF

Celeste Davis   (serves 4)
Delicious on salads! Mix with avocado or use as a dip with raw veggies.

Ingredients
>   ¼ onion, diced
>   2 garlic cloves, minced
>   ½ jalapeno pepper, minced***
>   2 large tomatoes, chopped
>   2 Tablespoons cilantro, chopped (optional)
>   ½ fresh lime (juiced)
>   Celtic Sea Salt

Instructions

Combine all of the above, add Celtic Sea Salt to taste. Can also be made in a blender or food processor, just process each vegetable separately then mix together in a bowl. Store covered in the refrigerator for 3-5 days.

*** Do not touch the jalapeno with your hands; it is best to . wear gloves and be sure to wash your hands well when finished. The jalapeno juice will burn your skin or your eyes if you touch your eyes after touching the jalapeno. Hotness is in the juice and white membrane.

Spinach Pesto GF, SF, BF

Celeste Davis (makes approximately 1 cup)
No one will ever know it's not all basil!

Ingredients
>   ½ cup extra virgin olive oil
>   1-½ cups baby spinach, stems removed
>   ¾ cup fresh basil leaves
>   ½ cup walnuts or pine nuts (soak first)

Spinach Pesto continued

6 oz. raw Sharp white cheese, grated, or raw Parmesan (Parmesan Reggiano)

3 large garlic cloves, peeled and quartered

Instructions

Use your S blade in your food processor. Combine 2 Tablespoons of the olive oil, the spinach, basil, nuts, cheese and garlic. Run food processor until nearly smooth, stopping processor, scrape down sides as needed. Drizzle in remaining olive oil until mixture is smooth. Store in sealed glass container and refrigerate for 1-2 days or freeze for 1 month, thaw and use immediately. Excellent stirred into pasta, on sandwiches or pizza or as an appetizer on toasted bread.

MARINADES

Spicy Lemon Marinade GF, DF, NSO, BF

Robb Davis
Delicious marinade for grilled or roasted veggies, meats, as stir-fry sauce.

Ingredients

4 Tablespoons fresh lemon juice

3 Tablespoons rice vinegar

3 Tablespoons Braggs Raw Apple Cider Vinegar

3 Tablespoons cold pressed extra virgin olive oil

2 Tablespoons extra virgin unrefined coconut oil

3 Tablespoons Braggs Amino Acids or wheat free tamari

3 Tablespoons raw honey

2 Tablespoons minced organic garlic

1 ½ Tablespoons chili pepper flakes

1 Tablespoon grated ginger

1/3 yellow onion, chopped fine in food processor

Spice Lemon Marinade Instructions continued
Combine in all ingredients in magic bullet or food processor, season with Celtic Sea Salt and white pepper to taste. Store in sealed glass jar in refrigerator for up to 10 days.

Tasty Teriyaki Sauce GF, DF, NSO, BF

Celeste Davis (makes about 3 cups)
Use as a stir fry sauce, barbeque sauce, topping for veggie burgers, serve with quinoa or brown rice, dip for rice paper wraps.

Ingredients
- ½ cup Raw Agave Nectar
- 2 cups Braggs Amino Acids(or gluten free soy sauce)
- 8 green onions, cut into 1 ½ inch pieces
- 4 slices fresh ginger, peeled
- 1-3 garlic cloves, minced
- ¼ cup pineapple or fresh orange juice
- ½ cup raw honey

Instructions
Combine all but raw honey in saucepan. Bring to boil. Mixture will foam, stir and when double in size, remove from heat. Stir in raw honey. Use in place of teriyaki sauce for BBQ, stir fry, etc. Store refrigerated in a sealed glass jar for up to 3 weeks.

Tropical Marinade GF, DF, NSO, BF

Celeste Davis (makes about 2 cups)
Excellent on grilled veggies, chicken, fish, as a stir-fry sauce.

Ingredients
- ½ cup coconut oil, olive oil or Grape seed oil
- ½ cup lemon or lime juice
- ¼ cup filtered water

Tropical Marinade continued
¼ cup organic Dijon mustard
2 Tablespoons raw local honey or raw agave nectar
2 Tablespoons minced garlic
2 Tablespoons chopped fresh basil leaves
½ teaspoon Celtic Sea Salt
½ teaspoon fresh ground white pepper or red pepper flakes

Instructions
Blend Ingredients together in magic bullet, food processor or blender.

Coconut Oil is solid oil at room temperature. To create the marinade you must melt the coconut oil in a pan of water on the stovetop. Re-warm the marinade slightly to use. The coconut oil gives an amazing flavor.

Asian Salsa GF, DF, NSO, BF

Celeste Davis
This AMAZING sweet and spicy sauce is fabulous on lettuce wraps, or as a dipping sauce for rice paper wraps. Also a great salad dressing with green onion, mandarin oranges and sliced almonds. Personally, I could put it in a cup and drink it!
Ingredients
1/8 to ¼ cup raw local honey
½ cup filtered water
2 Tablespoons Braggs Amino Acids (no-MSG soy sauce OR gluten free soy sauce if needed)
2 Tablespoons rice wine vinegar
2 Tablespoons organic ketchup
1 Tablespoon fresh lemon juice

Asian Salsa continued
        1/8 teaspoon toasted sesame oil
        1 Tablespoon hot mustard (Asian style)
        2 teaspoons filtered water
        1-2 teaspoon minced garlic
        1-2 teaspoons red chili paste

Instructions
Mix well in magic bullet or with a wire whip. Store in sealed
glass jar refrigerator for up to 5 days.

CHAPTER 12 RAW VEGGIES AND SALADS

A healthy lifestyle requires 50% to 75% of your food be from raw fruits and vegetables every day. Make two or three raw salads on your prep day and your meals will be a snap!

If I were Queen I would decree that EVERYONE in my kingdom eat a raw Kale salad every day! Kale is THE most nutritious veggie there is and all the Kale salad recipes in this book are easy and delicious.

The Apple Annie's and the Garlicky Kale salads are very popular. In fact, they demonstrated the Apple Annie's on the store floor and people come in months later to ask for the recipe.

You really don't need a recipe for a tasty raw salad, just look in the refrigerator and pull out some of your favorite veggies, chop them to the size you enjoy, add your favorite salad dressing, toss well and you have just created a new recipe!

Two veggie sandwich ideas are also in this section. The recipes in this section are favorites from our Whole Foods cooking classes. We use them regularly as well.

Aunt Celeste's Kale Salad GF, DF, NSO, HF, HP, BF

Celeste Davis (makes about 4-5 cups)
Believe it or not, this is one of our all-time favorite recipes. People tell me they take it to potlucks and dinners with all the unhealthy food and people rave about it and ask for the recipe!

Ingredients

    1 bunch of Kale, washed, remove stems and tear into chunks

    2 fresh, crisp apples like Gala or Honey Crisp

    ½ sweet yellow onion or red onion (if it is super strong smelling, use less)

    1/3 cup raw, soaked sunflower seeds or raw pumpkin seeds

    1/3 cup organic, no sugar raisins, or dried cranberries or cherries

    2 Tablespoons fresh lemon juice

    1 Tablespoon Braggs Raw Apple Cider Vinegar

    1-teaspoon Celtic Sea Salt

    2 Tablespoons grape seed oil or olive oil

Instructions

In your Food Processor with the S blade. Put apple chunks and onion pieces together, pulse a few times until a coarse chop, and remove to a large bowl. Put kale in FP, filling FP bowl to top but not packed. Pulse kale 10 times or until fine chop (not liquefied). Remove chopped kale and do again until all kale is chopped. Put kale in bowl with apples and onion, add 1 teaspoon of Celtic Sea Salt.

Squeeze or massage with your hands a few times to break down the fiber of the kale and rub the Celtic Sea Salt into the kale. (Approximately 10-15 massages).

Add lemon juice, vinegar, oil and raisins, and sunflower or pumpkin seeds. Stir Well. Seal and store in fridge for up to 5 days. Will improve as time goes by as the kale softens and flavors blend.

Garlicky Kale Salad GF, DF, NSO, HF, HP, BF

Celeste Davis (makes about 4 cups)
Alternate your Kale salads between this one and Apple Annie's for great variety. You don't need a food processor for this one!

Ingredients
    1 bunch Kale
    Braggs Amino Acids (no MSG soy sauce)
    1 head roasted garlic
    1 Tablespoon lemon juice
    4 Tablespoons Grape seed Veganaise
    1 Tablespoon fresh dill
    Grated White Pepper to taste
    3 Tablespoons Raw pumpkin seeds

Instructions

Wash Kale, remove stem, tear into bite sized pieces and put in a large bowl.. Add 1-2 teaspoons Braggs Amino Acids to Kale. Using your hands, mix, stir, and squeeze kale, kind of like a light massage, so the Braggs Amino Acids are on the Kale leaves. Massage just enough so the Kale is not so hard and grass-like.

Put the garlic, lemon juice, Grape seed Veganaise, dill and white pepper into your magic bullet or food processor and blend until smooth. Pour the dressing over the Kale and stir well. Stir in raw pumpkin seeds. Store covered in refrigerator for up to 3 days.

Kale Puttanesca Fresca GF, NSO, HF, HP, BF

Celeste Davis (serves 6)
This is a wonderful pasta/fresh veggie salad that features the nutrition giant Kale! Even your non-healthy eaters will enjoy it. If you are making a batch to eat all week, cook the pasta when you make the salad but just add the pasta right before serving it so the pasta doesn't get mushy.

Kale Puttanesca Fresca Ingredients

    1 box Quinoa penne pasta (GLUTEN FREE)
    2 pounds fresh tomatoes (or canned San Marzano)
    1 box cherry tomatoes (or grape)
    1 medium zucchini squash
    1 head lacinto kale (remove heavy stem)
    3 cloves fresh garlic
    ¼ cup fresh basil leaves
    ¼ cup fresh parsley leaves
    2 sprigs fresh oregano
    1 teaspoon – 1 Tablespoon chili pepper flakes
    3-4 Tablespoons olive oil (first cold press, Mediterranean)
    20 pitted kalamata olives
    3 Tablespoons capers
    2 ounces Coarse grated or shaved Parmesan reggiano (raw parmesan)
    Celtic Sea Salt & Ground White Pepper to taste

Instructions

For an extra garlic punch, rub serving bowl with one clove of garlic, set aside. Prepare penne pasta according to package directions, cool. Grate or shave Parmesan reggiano (raw parmesan).

Chop tomatoes in bite sized pieces

Using the Slicing Blade of your food processor, thin slice onion & kale (roll several pieces of kale in a long tube and put the thicker end in first. Use the Shredding Blade of your food processor to shred zucchini. Use the S blade of your food processor, to pulse to fine chop basil, fresh basil, oregano and parsley. Combine all with tomatoes, olive oil, olives, and capers. Stir in pasta. Sprinkle with Parmesan cheese just before serving. Serve at room temperature.

Asian Sprout Salad GF, DF, NSO, HF, HP, BF

Celeste Davis (serves 4)
Sprouts have from 100 to 300 times the nutrition of the full plant.
This is an unusual but delicious salad. Serve on top of finely shredded
green cabbage or bok choy. Don't like bean sprouts, substitute raw
cashews or sliced almonds.

Ingredients

> 1 lb. mung bean sprouts (raw or you can poach for ½
> to 2 minutes)
> 1 cup cucumber, peeled & sliced
> ½ cup grated carrot
> 1 cup sweet pepper (any or all colors), chopped
> ½ head green cabbage or bok choy cut into chunks
> Any other veggies you like
> Mandarin orange slices

Instructions

Put mung bean sprouts in large bowl. Peel 1-large carrot and
1 large cucumber.

Using slicing blade of food processor, slice cucumber and
sweet pepper, put in bowl with mung bean sprouts. Using
same slicing blade, slice cabbage, put in a separate bowl (this
is the base of the salad). Using grating blade of food
processor, grate carrot. Slice, grate or chop any veggies you
want to add.

Mix all veggies together except cabbage or bok choy and stir
in Nutty Asian Sweet & Hot Dressing in Chapter 11, until all
veggies are well covered. Serve over fine shredded cabbage.
or bok choy.

Broccoli Salad GF, DF, NSO, HF, HP, BF

Celeste Davis (serves 4)
My version of the popular salad bar and potluck salad.; this is a great every day salad as well.

Ingredients
    4 cups broccoli florets
    Peeled and sliced broccoli stems
    ¾ cup Grape seed Veganaise
    2 Tablespoons raw honey
    2 Tablespoons fresh lemon juice
    ¼ cup raw sunflower seeds
    ½ cup organic raisins

Instructions
Cut the stems off the broccoli and peel the thick outer part away.

In food processor, using the S blade, coarse chop broccoli florets and stems with a few pulses.

Make a dressing with Veganaise, honey or agave nectar, and lemon juice. Add sunflower seeds and raisins and stir well, pour over broccoli and stir well. Refrigerate for 1-2 hours before serving for flavors to blend. Store in sealed glass container in refrigerator for 3-5 days.

Quick Asian Broccoli Salad GF, DF, NSO, HF, HP, BF

Celeste Davis (serves 4) inspired by recipe from Kathleen Phillips
Ingredients
    ½ cup soaked almonds, sliced or coarse chopped
    1 12 oz. package broccoli slaw or 3 cups shredded broccoli stem or angel hair cabbage
    1 12 oz package mixed broccoli, broccoli slaw and snow peas
    ¼ cup thin sliced red onion or green onion

Quick Asian Broccoli Salad continued
1 cup shredded carrots
1 recipe Asian Salad Dressing Chapter 11

Instructions
Mix all veggies together in a large container. Stir in Almonds. Toss in Asian Salad Dressing. Top with sesame seeds.

Tips
Will keep for 3 days, but it's best when fresh. You can peel the tough outer covering off the broccoli stem and run through your food processor with the shredding blade, very nutritious! Add other veggies you have on hand.

Aunt Pauline's Cucumber and Tomato Salad GF, DF, NSO, HF, BF

Celeste Davis(serves 4-6)
Aunt Pauline's garden always provided most of our summer meals when I went to visit. "Go get some tomatoes and cucumbers from the garden, and grab a pinch of dill too." "And remember to shut the gate so the dog doesn't get in the garden!"
This salad is definitely best as a fresh-out-of-the-garden salad when cucumbers and tomatoes are in season. Add some raw Feta cheese or 4 ounces of grilled chicken just before serving....love those summer time veggies!

Ingredients
1 Tablespoon extra virgin olive oil
3 Tablespoons fresh lemon juice
½ teaspoon Celtic Sea Salt
1/3 teaspoon freshly ground white pepper
½ teaspoon raw local honey
3-4 garden fresh organic tomatoes
1 large organic fresh cucumber
1 Tablespoon fresh dill
Optional add grilled chicken, feta or blue cheese

<< CHEF'S TOMATO TIPS: Always sharpen your knife before and after cutting tomatoes. Tomato skins create dull knife blades! >>

Instructions
In a large bowl, combine oil, lemon juice, Celtic Sea Salt, pepper, and or honey. Stir well.

Cut tomatoes in wedges and thin slice cucumber and red onion.

Add tomatoes, cucumber and red onion to dressing,; toss well and refrigerate. When ready to serve, add dill and cheese or chicken and toss again.

DID YOU SHUT THE GARDEN GATE?

Jicama Salad GF, DF, NSO, HF, BF

Celeste Davis, (serves 4)
You should really try this salad. Jicama is a cool, crisp and somewhat sweet and crunchy delight! Looks like a smooth skinned coconut, has the texture of a radish with a sweet and watery flavor.
Ingredients
> 1 large Jicama, peeled and cut into thin strips or shredded
> 2 large carrots, peeled and cut into thin strips or shredded
> 1-cup thin sliced red onion
> ½ of each of these peppers (use organic) red, green, yellow or orange

Jicama Salad Instructions Continued
Peel brown skin off Jicama with potato peeler.

Use S Blade in Food Processor and Shred Jicama and carrots, put in large bowl. Use slicing blade in Food Processor and thin slice red onion. Top with Creamy Lime dressing in Chapter 11. Serve on a bed of spring mix or baby spinach.

Rice Paper Wraps GF, DF, NSO, HF

Celeste Davis
Like a salad –to-go or serve as an appetizer with an Asian meal. Our friend Vui from Whole Foods in Franklin, TN taught us this favorite food of her native home in South Vietnam. Vui said when she was growing up the teenagers would sit around and munch on these in the same way American teens munch on chips and candy.
Imagine your teenagers sitting around a bowl of filtered water, piles of fresh herbs and veggies, making rice paper wraps....try it, they may love it!

Ingredients
> Rice Paper from Asian section of grocery (these cannot be cooked, must use raw like this)
> Variety of your favorite fresh herbs
> Fresh baby spinach or spring mix
> Your choice of thinly sliced raw veggies such as cucumbers, avocado, carrots, green
> Onions
> Nut pate or hummus

Instructions
Dip rice paper into bowl of filtered water for 1-3 seconds

Put on a cutting board, careful not to wrinkle. Put some spinach or spring mix and veggies on the top of the rice paper. Top it with some fresh herbs. Roll away from you like a burrito, folding in the edges. Cut in half to serve. Serve with a dip or dressing like Asian Salsa in Chapter 11.

Rice Paper Wraps Example
* 1 Rice Paper Wrap
* 5 Baby Spinach leaves

- 1 Sprig Fresh Basil
- 1 Sprig Fresh Dill
- 1 Sprig Fresh Mint
- 1 teaspoon Grated Carrots
- 1 teaspoon Grated Zucchini
- 1 thin Avocado slice

Check out our rice paper wraps video on you tube
http://youtu.be/1ik7v4jarhg

Green Goddess Sandwich GF, DF, SF, BF

Celeste Davis

The morning after a Whole Foods cooking class, 11-year-old Alyssa recently said, "Mom can we go by Whole Foods and pick up the sprouted grain bread so we can make those yummy Green Goddess sandwiches?"

Many share her sentiments. You will not miss the meat because the spinach gives the texture of meat. All the veggies and the Green Goddess spread make it fabulously fresh and light.

Green Goddess Sandwich Ingredients & Instructions
- 1-2 slices Sprouted Grain Bread, like Alvarado or Ezekiel bread, or a spelt wrap.
- Top bread with Green Goddess dressing, to taste
- 2 inches of baby spinach
- Thinly sliced red onion, cucumber, tomato and avocado.

Three minute Salad GF, DF, NSO, HF, BF

Celeste Davis serves 4

This is a weekly staple at our house, different dressings give the veggies different flavors. Make one up each week to serve with your 2 handfuls of greens.

Ingredients
1 bag of cut up raw veggies – broccoli, cauliflower, carrots
Any other raw veggies you enjoy – onions, peppers, celery, radishes, beets

Instructions

Mix with Sweet and Sour dressing in Chapter 11 or your favorite organic, dairy free dressing. Store in a glass container, will keep up to 3 days

GREEN SALADS

Garlic Spinach Salad   GF, NSO, HF, HP, BF

Celeste Davis

The Roasted Garlic Dressing is much like warm bacon dressing but without the toxic pig fat! This is a great companion for any main dish.

Ingredients

    1 lb. fresh spinach

    ¼ red onion, sliced thin

    2 oz. raw goat cheese, broken into chunks

    Roasted Garlic Dressing in Chapter 11

Garlic Spinach Salad Instructions

Toss spinach and onion with Roasted Garlic Dressing, sprinkle cheese on top. Serve immediately. This salad does not keep well after dressing has been added.

Spinach Poppy Seed Salad GF, NSO, HF, HP, BF

Celeste Davis

This is a refreshing and quick salad in a meal.

Ingredients

    1 lb. fresh spinach, washed & dried

    1 pint strawberries, washed & halved

    ¼ Red Onion, thinly sliced

    1/2 cup pecan halves, soaked first and then toasted

    2 oz. raw goat cheese (feta)

Instructions

Toss spinach, strawberries, cheese and hot pecans in Berry Lemon Poppy Seed dressing in Chapter 11. The hot nuts will slightly wilt the greens. Salad does not store well, serve immediately. Make it healthier by eliminating the cheese and adding a few more nuts!

<< Are you getting enough leafy green veggies? Each person should have FOUR handfuls of leafy greens per day!

How to get them in? Add Spinach to your smoothie and eat one or more of these salads each day!

Make your portion a BIG handful! >>

Harvest Time Green Salad GF, NSO, HF, HP, BF

Celeste Davis (serves one person)
A wonderful lunchtime favorite when the apples and pears are freshly harvested.

Ingredients

> 2 handfuls of leafy greens
> 1 slice of red onion
> ½ organic fresh crop apple, chopped(honey crisp is our favorite)
> ½ organic ripe pear, chopped
> 1-2 Tablespoons raw feta or blue cheese
> 1 Tablespoon Toasted Pecans or Walnuts
> Crunchy Pumpkin Seed Topping Chapter 15
> Cranberry Vinaigrette

Instructions

Combine all and serve. You can make ahead if you do not put dressing on. Make it healthier by eliminating the cheese and adding a few more nuts!

Sushi Salad GF, DF, NSO, HF, HP, BF

By Celeste Davis serves 4-6
Everything but the seaweed and the rice!
This is a beautiful salad to take to a party or serve to guests but it is also very good to make just for you! Amounts of salad Ingredients depend on how many you are serving, adjust accordingly.
Do a taste-test on the dressing with the ginger and the brown mustard and the Braggs Amino Acids, to your preference.   The dressing will keep for several days in the fridge.

Ingredients

> Your favorite greens (no iceberg lettuce)
> 1 ripe but not mushy avocado, halved & sliced thin
> 1 Cucumber sliced thin
> ½ Red Onion sliced thin
> Grilled salmon (can be hot or cold)
> 1 recipe Orange Ginger Vinaigrette dressing in Chapter 11

Instructions

Toss greens and veggies in Orange Ginger Vinaigrette dressing and top with salmon and avocado. To make it beautiful, toss greens just before serving and arrange cucumber, onion, avocado and salmon on top. Make it better...top with Crunchy Quinoa.

Tropical Salad   GF, NSO, HF, BF

Celeste Davis
Refreshing fruit salad to add to your 2 handfuls of greens, add some grilled chicken, chick peas or lima beans and enjoy!
Ingredients

> 1 avocado, cubed
> 8 pineapple chunks, cubed
> 1 papaya or mango, cubed
> ½ celery stalk, diced
> ½ cup mango or pineapple juice, unsweetened

Instructions

Coarse chop pineapple, mango and celery with your S blade in your Food Processor. Juice ½ cup pineapple in your juicer. Combine all and serve over mixed greens.

Janice's Asian Citrus Pasta Salad   GF, DF, NSO, HF, HP, BF

Modified by Celeste Davis   (serves 4 as a main dish, more as a side dish)
This is an adaptation of a favorite salad made by my good friend Janice Gietzen. A Whole Foods cooking class favorite this is a great salad to take to a party or serve to guests; however, it is also very good to make just for you! Amounts of salad Ingredients depend on how many you are serving, adjust accordingly.
Cook pasta and marinate veggies the day before, toss together just before serving.

Ingredients

> 1 package small penne pasta (Quinoa or Rice Pasta is best, gluten free)
> 1 bunch asparagus
> 2 large carrots
> ¼ lb. Snow peas or Snap Peas
> 1 lb. broccoli florets
> 1 small Vidalia onion
> 2 cups garbanzo beans or fresh green peas
> ¼ cup Better Than Teriyaki Sauce or (Veri Teriyaki Sauce at most grocery stores)
> ¼ cup orange juice

Janice's Asian Citrus Pasta Salad Instructions

Make it raw by putting veggies in marinade one day in advance, they will soften as if they were steamed.

OR Steam veggies very lightly (just to warm to touch). Toss veggies in approximately ½ cup Better Than Teriyaki Sauce or use Veri Teriyaki Sauce.

Cook pasta according to package directions. Toss all Ingredients together, add more sauce as needed to taste.

**Non-vegan version: Sauté sliced free range chicken or turkey in a little Grape seed oil, add teriyaki sauce, simmer, then add veggies and pasta, serve warm or cold.

*<< **Health Tip!**: Remember to keep your animal protein to less than 12 ounces per week.*

Use raw or toasted nuts and seeds or cooked beans for protein on salads. >>

CHAPTER 13   COOKED VEGGIES

Make 25% of your daily veggies cooked, eat the rest raw!

The SAD (standard American diet) way of making veggies is to smother their flavor, beautiful color and texture with some kind of heavy, usually creamy, fatty or cheesy sauce.

The recipes in this section use delicious, aromatic, healing herbs to compliment, not conceal, the wonderful flavors and textures of vegetables.

When using herbs, fresh is always best. If you use dried herbs, use them up within 3 months, they lose their flavor if kept longer.

If using fresh herbs you will need to use more in quantity than dried. 1 Tablespoon of fresh or 1 teaspoon of dried is a good rule to remember.

Recipes generally add herbs towards the end of the cooking time to retain their fresh flavor.

Remember, while cooked veggies have vitamins and minerals, the healing powerhouse enzymes are killed by heat above 118 degrees F. Be sure and eat more raw veggies than cooked.

Grilled Veggies GF, DF, NSO, HF, BF

Celeste Davis (serves 4)
Make extra, these are great hot or cold!

Ingredients

    2 med carrots
    2 large yellow bell peppers quartered, and seeded
    1 large red onion quartered with root intact to hold slices together while grilling
    2 med red potatoes, boiled and just slightly undercooked, then slice in ¼ inch slices
    1 small fennel bulb, washed, long stems removed but with root intact (save feathery leaves)
    1 small zucchini sliced
    1 Tablespoon Grape seed oil
    Celtic Sea Salt
    Fresh ground white pepper or crushed red pepper flakes

Instructions-Heat the grill to med temp.

Peel carrots and slice into thick slices. Blanch by dropping in boiling filtered water for 3-4 minutes, then put in cold water. Keep boiling carrot water and cook potatoes for about 5 minutes, then cool and slice into ¼ inch slices. Quarter the onions but leave the root intact to hold the onion together. Remove the feathery part of the fennel, set aside for later, cut fennel bulb in half or quarters, leaving the root intact. Slice zucchini in about ½ inch rounds or chunks.

Toss veggies in about 2 Tablespoons of Grape seed oil or coconut oil and season with Celtic Sea Salt and pepper.

Place veggies on the grill and cook until they are the desired tenderness, about 2 minutes per side, and lightly brown. DO NOT CHAR. If the veggies begin to brown faster than they are cooking, raise the grill higher above the heat, move the veggies to a cooler area of the grill or transfer to a platter until the grill temperature is lower.

Sweet Potato Fries with Rosemary GF, DF, HF, BF

Celeste Davis (Serves 6) Low fat & healthy version.

Ingredients

> 2 lbs. sweet potatoes
> 1 teaspoon Grape seed oil
> 1 teaspoon lemon juice
> 1 teaspoon dried rosemary

Instructions preheat oven to 375 degrees F

Wash and cut sweet potatoes into sticks or wedges.

Place potatoes in a bowl and toss with oil, then spread out onto a baking sheet and sprinkle with rosemary. Bake about 30 minutes at 375° degrees F, or until browned and tender. You may want to turn potatoes over half way through baking time. Sprinkle with lemon juice.

Yukon Gold Oven Fries GF, DF, HF, BF

Celeste Davis (serves one; add half to one potato per person)
Michael Pollen stated in his book Food Rules, it's Ok to eat junk food from time to time as long as you make it yourself. These oven fries are fabulous and have nutritional benefits if you use organic Yukon Gold potatoes. There is a vast difference in the fiber and nutritional value of non-organic potatoes, they are not worth the calories. Always use organic.

Ingredients

> 1 organic Yukon Gold potato, the size of the palm of your hand
> 1 teaspoon Grape seed oil
> Celtic Sea Salt and Crushed Red Pepper to taste

Instructions Preheat oven to 450 degrees
Put the pan you are going to cook the potatoes on in the oven while you prepare the fries, this will help to put a nice brown color on your fries

Wash outside of potato well. Cut potato into strips by cutting it in half length wise and then cut each half in half or thirds diagonally, slice into the size of fries you like. Soak the potato slices in water for 15 minutes if you can, if you don't have that much time, rinse them well and roll them in a paper towel or towel to pat dry. This helps to eliminate excess starch.

Toss potatoes in Grape seed oil and spread on pre-heated pan; don't overcrowd pan.

Bake in oven for 10 minutes on the bottom shelf, just over the element.

Remove from the oven, turn the fries over so the other side is in contact with the hot pan and bake another 10 minutes.

Yukon Gold Oven Fries are baked when nicely browned on each side and tender in the middle. Non organic potatoes are not healthy. A good potato will produce a crispy brown crust.

Serve with ORGANIC KETCHUP or any other toppings you enjoy.

<< *Conventional Ketchup and Relish are primarily made of High Fructose Corn Syrup. Only buy organic ketchup and relish.*

Words that mean High Fructose Corn Syrup

Corn Syrup, Corn Sweetener, Maltose, Maltodextrin

222

I'm sure there will be more "code words" for high fructose corn syrup as wise consumers are beginning to reject products with high fructose corn syrup. >>

Sweet Orange Stir Fry GF, DF, NSO, HF, HP, BF

Celeste Davis (Serves 4)
This a delicious Asian vegetarian dish. It has several steps but your food processor makes it quick. Make it a lettuce wrap by chopping your veggies smaller with the S blade and wrapping it in a romaine lettuce leaf! Top with "Asian Salsa", recipe in Chapter 11. PF Yum!

Sauce Ingredients
> 3 Tablespoons Raw Agave Nectar
> 6 Tablespoons fresh squeezed orange juice
> 1-Tablespoon Braggs Amino Acids
> 1 teaspoon toasted Sesame oil
> 1 Tablespoon non-GMO cornstarch or arrow root
> ¼ to ½ teaspoon red pepper flakes

Stir Fry Ingredients
> ¾ cup raw cashews
> 1-teaspoon sesame oil
> 1 red bell pepper
> 1 cup of green veggies (green beans, broccoli, zucchini)
> 1 sweet onion
> 1 large carrot
> 2 stalks celery
> 1-inch ginger, fresh
> 3 garlic cloves or 1 Tablespoon minced

Precooking Prep
Run 2-3 sweet, juicing oranges, (Valencia is my favorite) through your juicer, to make 6 Tablespoons (about ½ a cup) of orange juice. Combine Sauce Ingredients in a small bowl.

In Your Food Processor
Using slicing blade slice onion, celery, carrots, put in a bowl

Using same blade (don't clean out the bowl) slice peppers and green veggies.

With a Hand Grater

Mince Garlic. Mince ginger with fine grater.

Stir Fry

In a dry skillet, toast cashews over medium heat about 3 minutes until lightly toasted. Watch continually because nuts burn really fast. Set aside in a bowl.

In same skillet sauté onion, celery, pepper and veggies in 1 Tablespoon Grape seed or coconut oil about 2 minutes. You may need to do this in batches if your skillet is small.

Add 1 Tablespoon Grape seed or coconut oil, ginger, garlic and red pepper flakes, cook 1 more minute.

Stir in 2 Tablespoons filtered water and cashews; cook until veggies are crunchy tender.

Sauce

Combine orange juice and cornstarch, mix well. Pour over veggie mixture, and stir again. Bring to simmer, stir again and remove from heat. Stir when serving. Serve with Quinoa or Brown Rice.

How To Cook Winter Squash GF, DF, NSO

Celeste Davis
For Acorn, Spaghetti, Butternut, Pumpkin and other hard winter squash.
Squash is hard to cut. To make it easier, put whole squash in oven at 375 degrees F for 10-15 minutes, then cut in half, length wise.

Scoop out seeds, save seeds to roast. Rub or spray flesh of squash with Grape seed oil   Put cut side down on a baking pan or cookie sheet. **Bake** rind side up about 30 to 40 minutes at 375 degrees F. or **Boil** 20 minutes or so.

Spaghetti Squash
Separate strands of spaghetti squash by running a fork through the squash "from stem to stern".   Use cooked spaghetti squash in place of spaghetti noodles in the Spaghetti Squash Primavera recipe or in place of crab in the "Faux Crab Cakes" recipe.

Acorn, Butternut, pumpkin and other hard winter squashes
Scoop out "flesh" and mash or cut into chunks.   Try the Butternut Squash Soup or the Pineapple Acorn Squash recipes in this chapter.

Cooked winter and spaghetti squash can be frozen in small portions in Ziploc brand freezer bags for about one month. Write the date on the freezer bag.

<< Winter Squash Is A Nutritional Powerhouses! High in fiber, vitamin C, carotenes, B-vitamins, potassium

Pumpkin seeds are anti-parasitic and are known to help reduce the symptoms of benign prostatic hyperplasia (prostate). >>

Roasted Pumpkin or Squash Seeds GF, DF, SF, HF, HP, BF
Celeste Davis (makes one to two cups)
Instructions
Preheat oven to 350 degrees F. (or see below for lower slower method).

1) Clean the pulp off the pumpkin seeds (or squash seeds), and dry with paper towels.

2) If desired, toss with a little Grape seed oil. You only need enough to barely coat, otherwise, they will be greasy. Add Celtic Sea Salt and any kind of seasoning you want - garlic powder, Cajon seasoning, dried chili powder, Celtic Sea Salt, or whatever sounds good to you!

3) Cover a baking sheet with parchment paper and spread the seeds out in one layer.

Bake for 3-5 minutes, until seeds just start to color and are fragrant. Sometimes I use a longer but safer method of a lower temperature. If you roast the seeds at 250 degrees F., you don't have to watch them as carefully. It takes about 45 - 60 minutes.

Pineapple Acorn Squash GF, DF, NSO, HF, BF

Celeste Davis (serves 4-6)
Even the kids love this sweet comfort food, make two and freeze one.
Ingredients
> 1 large acorn squash, precooked
> ½ cup fresh pineapple
> 1 -2 cloves fresh garlic or 1 teaspoon garlic powder
> 1 Tablespoon Grape seed oil
> 1 teaspoon cinnamon
> ¼ teaspoon cloves
> ½ teaspoon Celtic sea salt
> ground white pepper

While squash is cooking, puree ½ cup of fresh pineapple in a blender or food processor using S blade. Add 1-2 cloves of garlic. Add 1 Tablespoon oil; coconut oil is my personal favorite but you can use Grape seed oil. Add salt, cinnamon, and cloves to taste.

Take squash out of oven, scoop squash out of shell with a spoon, mash to break up big pieces and place into baking dish. Pat down until even and cover with the pineapple garlic mixture. Bake at 350 degrees F for 15 minutes more.

Serve with a nice fresh salad. Can be refrigerated and eaten warm or cold later.

Cranberry/Pineapple Acorn Squash GF, DF, NSO, HF, BF

Celeste Davis (serves 4)
This is to die for! You can purchase frozen cranberries all year long.

Ingredients
- 1 large acorn squash, precooked
- 1 ½ cups fresh or frozen cranberries
- 1 Tablespoon raw Agave Nectar
- 1 Tablespoon filtered water
- 1 teaspoon cinnamon
- ¼ teaspoon cloves
- ½ teaspoon Celtic sea salt

Instructions
Pat acorn squash into a greased baking dish. Gently (on medium or low) Heat 1 ½ cups cranberries with 1Tablespoon raw Agave Nectar and 1Tablespoon filtered water until cranberries begin to pop open. Add Celtic sea salt, cinnamon and cloves to taste. Add cranberry mixture to pineapple mixture. Spread over Acorn Squash, reheat for 15 minutes at 350.

Spaghetti Squash GF, DF, NSO, HF, BF

Celeste Davis (serves 4)
Spaghetti Squash is a low carbohydrate and tasty alternative to regular pasta. Make extra and freeze for another time and to make the "Faux Crab Cakes". Keep in the freezer for up to 1 month.

PRIMAVERA SPAGHETTI SAUCE GF, DF, NSO

Celeste Davis (serves 4)
Ingredients
- 1 large sweet yellow onion
- 1 package baby bella mushrooms
- 1 medium zucchini
- 2 large cloves garlic (1 Tablespoon minced)

227

1 cup fresh green beans
1 jar organic or natural spaghetti sauce (we like
Newman's Sockarooni or Marinara sauce)

Instructions
Cook Spaghetti Squash see "How To Cook Winter Squash"
in this chapter.

While the squash is cooking make the sauce.

In Food Processor, using slicing blade, Slice onions,
mushrooms, zucchini, and garlic. Sauté onions, mushrooms,
zucchini and garlic slightly in 1-2 Tablespoons Grape seed oil.
Add organic Spaghetti Sauce and heat through. Serve over
cooked spaghetti squash or spelt or rice pasta. This would
also be good on a baked potato instead of butter and sour
cream. Top with some Parmesan Reggiano cheese.

Simmer to thicken and serve as a "ragout" with Faux Crab
Cakes.

Faux Crab Cakes   DF, HF, BF

Celeste Davis (makes 8-10 / 3-inch cakes)
*I LOVE crab cakes, but don't eat them due to the high levels of toxins.
In the Bible, God told His people not to eat shellfish and crustaceans.
He wasn't trying to be difficult or mean. God made shellfish,
crustaceans, and bottom fish to clean and filter the water they live in,
eating them is like having the contents of your vacuum cleaner for
dinner.*
*Enjoy this replacement that tastes like Crab Cakes. Top with a fruit
chutney, dip in organic cocktail sauce or salsa and serve with a nice
fresh salad.*

Ingredients
1½ cups cooked spaghetti squash
1 medium potato, boiled and cooled
1 cup zucchini shredded
2 garlic cloves

2 small colored peppers
1 small onion
1 cup organic bread crumbs or crushed organic
saltine crackers
¼ cup white Spelt flour
1 large egg 1 Tablespoon almond milk or whole
cream
1 teaspoon paprika
1 teaspoon Celtic sea salt
1 teaspoon parsley
2 Tablespoons Grape seed Veganaise
1 teaspoon Dijon mustard
Grape seed oil for frying

Instructions
Cook Spaghetti Squash see "How To Cook Winter Squash"
in this chapter.

You will need to sauté the veggies before you pan fry the crab
cakes. You can use the same pan or have 2 skillets available.

Prep Veggies
Using your shred blade shred zucchini, peppers, onion. Remove to
skillet that has 1 Tablespoon Grape seed oil in it. Shred cooled and
peeled potato, set aside.

In skillet
Sautee zucchini, garlic, onion, peppers in oil until tender, about 2
minutes. Add potato and spaghetti squash to zucchini mixture, and
remove from heat.

In Magic Bullet
Put bread or cracker crumbs in magic bullet cup, and add
spices and salt. Add egg, almond milk, Dijon mustard,
Veganaise. Blend well with magic bullet.

In Food Processor with S blade
Put all veggies in food processor, add egg mixture in magic
bullet and pulse 2 -3 times to blend well. Put mixture in a

bowl and cover. Refrigerate for 30 minutes or longer for mixture to become more solid and flavors to blend.

Cook the cakes
These cakes will be slightly thinner than the typical restaurant crab cakes.

Put 1-2 Tablespoons Grape seed oil in cast iron skillet, medium heat. Dip out ¼ to 1/3 cup with a measuring cup and gently drop onto the skillet, drop it CLOSE to the skillet so you don't splatter the oil. Use a spoon to form the mixture into a patty on the skillet, to the size and thickness you desire. Fry until crisp on one side, then turn and fry on other side. Cakes are done when they are firm and cooked in the middle. Drain on a paper towel, keep warm in the oven.

Vegan? Use 1 Tablespoon of finely ground flax seeds mixed with 2 Tablespoons filtered water to replace egg.

Add Protein by adding ¼ cup garbanzo beans to mixture.

Serve with left over Prima Vera sauce Roasted Red Pepper Vinaigrette or Tartar Sauce (recipe below).

TARTAR SAUCE: (keep in refrigerator for up to 1 week)
Put in magic bullet and blend:

> ¼ cup Veganaise
> 1 teaspoon Dijon mustard
> 2 Tablespoons Greek sliced pepperoncini peppers
> Juice from ¼ lime (Squeeze into bullet)
> 1/8 of a medium onion
> 1 clove garlic
> 2 inches fresh dill or ½ teaspoon dried dill

Veggie Kabobs GF, DF, NSO, HF, BF

Celeste Davis (serves 4)
Vegetables grill up nicely, make extra to eat cold or reheat in the oven.

Ingredients
1 of each:

Red Onion
Green Pepper
Yellow Pepper
Red Pepper
Zucchini
1 box Baby Bella Mushrooms
1 box grape or cherry tomatoes
1 recipe Tropical Marinade or purchase Veri Teriyaki Sauce
Bamboo Skewers

Put bamboo kabob skewers in filtered water to soak for one hour.

Make 1 recipe Tropical Marinade or purchase your favorite organic marinade.

Cut veggies in big chunks to go on skewers. Marinate Veggies in Tropical Marinade. If using Veri Teriyaki Sauce, dilute with ¼ cup lemon juice and ¼ cup water. Put veggies on skewer.

Roast in 450-degree oven for 10-15 minutes, check for tenderness. Veggies can also be put on grill for 2minutes per side, set a timer! Serve with quinoa and a big salad.

CHAPTER 14   "GOOD FOR YOU" SOUPS

Remember Grandma's Chicken Soup? Soups ave been used to heal for thousands of years. They are easy for the body to digest and are nutrient dense, the liquid is hydrating to the body.

Hippocrates, known as the father of medicine is quoted as saying "let food be your medicine and medicine be your food". This is the man that doctor's quote when they take their oath, stating they will do no harm. How far we have come! The healing soups are beneficial to people with degenerative disease, autoimmune disease and cancers.

> << CHEF'S TIP!: ADD A RICHER FLAVOR AND CREAMIER TEXTURE TO BROTH BASED SOUPS.

Remove some of the veggies from the broth. Onions, carrots, garlic, potatoes are especially good for this.

Cool the veggies slightly and blend to smooth in your magic bullet or blender. Stir blended veggies back into your soup. >>

Each soup is alkalizing and healing. Try not to use Celtic Sea Salt or any salt when allowing the body to heal.

Soups are also a quick and easy way to have a good nutritous meal ready after a busy day. You can even buy precut veggies and canned beans to "make it quicker".

All the soup recipes in this section make large portions. Serve some and freeze some for later or eat on it all week.

Soup is always great with a fresh salad, some warm or toasted bread and garlic butter or corn bread muffins.

HEALING SOUPS

Hippocrates Soup GF, DF, NSO, HF

Recipe for 1 person. This is used at Gerson Cancer clinics to restore cancer patients to health. It is also wonderful for sick children.
In a 2-quart pot put the following organic vegetables and cover with purified filtered water.

Ingredients

      1 medium celery knob (the end portion of the celery, cut off about 3-4 inches from bottom and wash well)

      *You can also use 3-4 stalks of celery instead of knob

      1 medium bunch of parsley

      2 small leeks, white part only

      2 medium onions

      1 handful of curly parsley

      3-4 tomatoes

      3-4 medium Yukon gold potatoes

      2-3 garlic cloves (use more if you love garlic)

Instructions

Scrub veggies well, do not peel.

Coarse chop with S blade or slice with slicing blade of food processor.

Hippocrates Soup Instructions Continued

Cook slowly for 3 hours, until soft, then blend well in a blender or food processor, blend until it is really pureed. Add salt sparingly after soup is cooked.

Use your cooking water and add until it reaches the soup-like texture you desire.

Let the soup cool before storing. Keep covered in refrigerator for no longer than 2-3 days.

Warm up as much as you will eat at a time, not the whole batch.

These soups restore minerals such as potassium & sodium.

Bieler Soup GF, DF, SF, HF

String beans are excellent for diabetics, to help heal the pancreas and lower blood sugar. For more health info, read **Food is Your Best Medicine: Dr. Bieler's Health Broth, and more** *by Henry Bieler and Maxine Block*

Ingredients
3 stalks celery, sliced
1 lb. organic string green beans
2 lbs. zucchini
Purified filtered water to cover veggies
1 handful of curly parsley

Instructions
Boil all veggies but parsley in filtered water until you can pierce with a fork. Drain veggies but reserve filtered water.

Puree the veggies and add your cooking water to desired taste and consistency. preference). Add parsely and blend well. You can also add: Carrots, Kale, Potatoes. Omit parsely for breastfeeding women as it can "dry up" milk.

Soups can be frozen and reheated on the stovetop! While they typically have a longer list of ingredients and more steps than other recipes, they are a quick way to have a healthy and delicious meal. We always have at least 2 varieties of soup in the freezer and generally make a fresh pot of something every week.

To make soup quick and easy, read through the recipe first. Chop your veggies in your food processor with the S blade for a coarse chop or the slicing blade for a prettier thin slice. To make it fast, buy your veggies already chopped from the grocery and just put it all together.

In Their Own Words

"My family loves the Easy 3 Bean Chili, we could live on it!"

"The dairy free Creamy Tomato Basil Soup is awesome! No one knew it was dairy free!"

"Phil's kitchen soup is a staple at our house and we serve it to guests, everyone loves it!"

"I didn't know I loved squash until I tried the creamy satisfying Butternut Squash Soup"

"The Quinoa Vegetable Soup was so easy to make, I used the veggies already cut up for salads and the soup was ready in no time!"

"15 Bean Soup is my husband's favorite; he is always so happy when he smells it cooking. It's a hearty, flavorful soup."

"Marvelous Minestrone is now my favorite soup, I love the slight Parmesan flavor without all the added fat from too much cheese."

Butternut Squash Soup GF, DF, NSO, HF, BF

Contributed by Sherri Hails (serves 6)
A Creamy Detox Favorite , this sweet and aromatic soup is fall in a cup! To learn how to cook a butternut squash see "How to Cook Winter Squash".

Ingredients and Instructions
Cook the veggies
Place face down on baking sheet:
> 1 Medium (3 lb) size butternut squash, Cut in half, remove seeds Squash will produce about 4 ½ cups of cooked squash.

Also put on the same baking sheet:
> 2 Carrots peeled
> 1/2 Vidalia Onion cut into Chunks
> 1 Zucchini, peeled & diced
> 1 Clove of Garlic chopped
> Drizzle all with Grape seed oil
> Cover with foil or a lid

Bake at 350 for 30-40 minutes

Scoop out Butternut Squash and put in a large pot add all the rest of the veggies and stir well.

Add:
> 1/2 teaspoon of ginger powder
> 1/2 teaspoon of cinnamon
> 1/2 teaspoon of curry powder
> A dash of Paprika
> 1/4 teaspoon of Nutmeg

Add:
> 2 Tablespoons Maple syrup
> 2 Tablespoons raw local honey
> 2 Tablespoons Braggs Raw Apple cider vinegar
> 2 Cups Organic Vegetable or chicken broth

Butternut Squash Soup Continued

Simmer for 20 minutes. If needed, add honey/ maple syrup/ curry/ ginger/ or Celtic Sea Salt & pepper to taste. Pour into blender or strain to puree. Add filtered water as needed for desired consistency. Enjoy!

3 Bean Easy Chili GF, DF, NSO, HF, HP, BF

Serves 4 Adapted from fatfreevegan.com Recipe by: Lisa Wood
This is a big detox favorite! Approximately 8 grams protein

Ingredients

    1 small onion chopped
    1 can organic red kidney beans, drained & rinsed
    1 can organic pinto chili beans in sauce do not drain
    1 can organic black beans, drained & rinsed
    1 can organic diced tomatoes
    2 cups organic V8-type juice (or make your own Spicy Tom, recipe
    ½ teaspoon garlic powder to taste
    1 teaspoon chili powder to taste
    ¼ teaspoon cumin powder taste

Instructions

Sauté the onion in a little filtered water instead of oil. Add the rest of Ingredients. Add more V8-type juice if you want the chili less thick. Adjust spices to taste. Simmer for about 10 minutes.

15 Bean Soup GF, DF, NSO, HF, HP, BF

Celeste Davis (16 one cup servings, 8-10 grams protein)
Don't let the long list of Instructions keep you from making this soup,
it is very simple, and the Instructions are detailed.
This is a very economical meal, one gallon of soup costs less than
$4.00 (25 cents per serving) if you have all the spices on hand. Notice
there is no fat in this recipe. Makes approximately 1 gallon of soup.
Eat some, freeze some.

Ingredients

One pound bag of 15 bean soup mix (throw away the seasoning packet....poison!)

½ bag of your favorite dry beans (for variety) (my favorite is butter beans, use your favorite)

1-2 medium sweet yellow onions

3-5 cloves of garlic

3 stalks of celery with the leaves (use the inside leaves of the celery)

1 small potato

1-15 ounce can organic Mexican style crushed tomatoes with jalapeno (if you like it spicy)

1 gallon filtered water

1 teaspoon crushed fennel seeds (whir in magic bullet or crush with a spoon, they won't be pulverized but it will release the flavor, just smash with the back of a spoon like you would a bug!)

1 Tablespoon (or to taste) chili powder

1 teaspoon ground cumin

1 teaspoon dried basil

¼ teaspoon crushed red pepper

White Pepper optional

<< CHEF'S TIP!: SERVE THIS CHILI STYLE SOUP WITH ORGANIC CORN BREAD AND CABBAGE SLAW.

Cost per serving about 25 cents! >>

15 Bean Soup Instructions continued

Soak The Beans: Wash the beans in a colander, remove any rocks (yes, folks, rocks) and dirt. Put in a very large pot or bowl and cover with filtered water to about 2-3 inches over the top of the beans. Cover the container of beans with a towel and leave on counter for 24 hours.

Prep The Veggies: Use your food processor, using the S blade (that is the one that looks like an S). Put large chunks of onion and celery and your cloves of garlic in the food processor bowl and pulse it (push, push, push), don't just turn it on or you will liquify the veggies. Pulse until they are a coarse chop, you know, little chunky pieces.

Wash the potato and cut it in half, the potato is in the beans to absorb some of the sugars that cause you to fluff when you eat them, after the beans are cooked you will throw it out (or you could give it to someone you don't and watch them fluff away!

Cook The Beans After the beans have soaked for 24 hours, transfer them to a sink full of cold filtered water, swish them around a few times with your hands to rinse well. Transfer them to a colander and drain; this will help to reduce gas from the beans when you eat them.

Put all beans in a big soup pot (or a crock pot) and cover with filtered water. The water should be about 2-4 inches above the beans, depending on whether you prefer a thin soup or a thicker one. I would start with less, you can always add more filtered water if it is too thick. DO NOT ADD CELTIC SEA SALT until beans are cooked, cooking beans with salt will make the beans tough. Add chopped onion and celery, potato and all spices.

15 Bean Soup Continued

Cook beans on the stove top or in the oven until they are tender and can be smashed with a spoon. About 2 hours at 350 degrees F or on a medium heat stove top. In a crock pot, turn them on medium or low and allow to cook for about 10 hours.

Soup is finished when beans are soft.

Remove potato (it also helps to reduce gas from beans).

Add more filtered water if you like it thinner.

Add Celtic Sea Salt to taste.

For a richer flavored broth add Better Than Boullion Vegetarian Vegetable Base. Start with one teaspoon, taste, stir and retaste. Add a little at a time until you like the flavor.

<< This stew like version would be good with a spinach salad, ranch dressing and garlic bread. >>

Adding Meat to Your Soup

If you put pork in this bean soup I will never speak to you again! It becomes immediately unhealthy when you add pork.

Purchase some chicken or turkey sausage for a smokey flavor, be sure and get the kind with no nitrites and no nitrates. You could also add ground turkey or some form of chicken.

You can purchase chicken and turkey sausages at Whole Foods either uncooked or cooked.

Changing The Flavor Of Your 15 Bean Soup:

You can use different types of beans and different flavors to change your soup.the first recipe is for a spicy chili type flavor. To make it a savory, stew-like flavor do the following:

Omit the chili powder, red pepper flakes and mexican style crushed tomatoes.

Add:

2 medium carrots, peeled and diced (throw them in the food processor with your onions and garlic)
2 stems of fresh rosemary or 1 teaspoon dry rosemary (if you use fresh, leave the rosemary on the stem, it will fall off as it cooks
8 fresh sage leaves or ½ teaspoon of dry sage, If you use fresh, thinly slice the sage leaves)
1 medium zucchini, diced
1 small bunch of kale or chard, trimmed of tough ends and veins and coarsely chopped (4 to 5 cups) Run the kale through your food processor, remember, pulse, pulse, and pulse. The finer the chop, the less anyone will notice it's in there!
1 14-ounce can petite diced tomatoes or chunky-style crushed tomatoes

Hearty Lentil Soup GF, DF, NSO, HF, HP, BF

Celeste Davis (serves 4)
Lentils are the most nutrient dense form of protein. 1 serving provides 7.9 grams of protein.

Ingredients

1 cup dried brown lentils
4 cups vegetable broth
1 (14 1/2 oz.) can diced tomatoes
2 tablespoons Grape seed oil
2 garlic cloves, diced

242

Hearty Lentil Soup continued
1 medium onion, diced
2 large carrots, peeled and sliced
2 celery stalks (including leaves,) chopped
1 bay leaf
2 tablespoons balsamic vinegar
Celtic Sea Salt and pepper to taste

Hearty Lentil Soup Instructions

Pour lentils in a bowl, cover with filtered water, and allow to sit overnight.

Over medium heat, cook onions in Grape seed oil in a large soup pan. Add garlic and celery. Once celery begins to soften, add carrots, tomatoes, bay leaf and vegetable stock.

Pour in drained lentils. Bring to a boil, reduce heat, and allow the soup to simmer for 30 minutes. Remove and discard bay leaf and add vinegar. Season with Celtic Sea Salt and red pepper flakes to taste.

Marvelous Minestrone GF, NSO, HF, HP, BF

Celeste Davis (serves 6-8, inspired by Rachel Ray)
This is a hearty, flavorful soup, packed with nutrition. , Don't let the long list of Ingredients scare you, your food processor makes it in a snap! Make this for company, eat some and freeze or eat on it all week long.
Ingredients
2 tablespoons expeller pressed extra-virgin olive oil
1/2 teaspoon crushed red pepper flakes
4 garlic cloves
3 portabella mushroom caps, chopped
2 medium onions, chopped
2 medium carrots, peeled and diced
2 celery ribs, chopped with greens
Celtic Sea Salt and freshly ground white pepper

Marvelous Minestrone Ingredients Continued

2 stems of fresh rosemary
8 fresh sage leaves, thinly sliced
1 medium zucchini, diced
1 small bunch of kale or chard, trimmed of tough ends and veins and coarsely chopped (4 to 5 cups)
2 15-ounce can Cannelloni beans, drained [also called white kidney beans]
1 14-ounce can petite diced tomatoes or chunky-style crushed tomatoes
1 quart organic chicken stock or broth made from **Better Than Bouillon Organic** Chicken Broth
2 cups vegetable stock or broth made from Better Than Bouillon Organic Vegetarian Vegetable broth
A piece of rind of raw Parmigianino Reggiano or goat cheese- buy a piece with the rind attached to it, cut from the outside of the wheel
1 cup Quinoa, Rinse and Soak for 15 minutes, rinse again

Instructions

Coarse chop all veggies in food processor with S blade. Rinse Quinoa, Soak for 15 minutes, rinse before adding to pot.

Heat a medium soup pot over medium-high heat and add the Grape seed oil. Add the red pepper flakes, garlic, mushrooms, onions, carrots, and celery. Cook for 5 to 6 minutes, until the mushrooms are lightly browned. Season with Celtic Sea Salt and white pepper and add the rosemary stems and the sage to the pot. [The rosemary will fall off the stem as it cooks.]

Add the zucchini and chopped greens and stir them into the pot until all the greens wilt down, 2 to 3 minutes. Add the beans, tomatoes, stocks and cheese rind. Place a lid on the pot and bring the soup to a boil. Uncover and add the soaked Quinoa. Cook the soup for 10-15 minutes at a rolling simmer, uncovered, until the Quinoa is transparent and tender. Remove the pot from the heat. Remove the rind and the bare rosemary stems (the leaves fall off into the soup as it cooks). Adjust the Celtic Sea Salt and white pepper to taste. Serve With: Homemade Sprouted Spelt Bread & Fresh Italian Salad.

Creamy Tomato Basil Soup   GF, DF, NSO, BF

Celeste Davis (serves 4)

This soup is delicious, rich and creamy with no dairy products, a cooking class favorite.

In 1973, the first meal I made for my boyfriend Phil, (now my husband) would have made my Home Economics teacher proud. It was so colorful and well balanced; Phil ate it right up, said it was wonderful and made ME proud. The appetizer was homemade cream of tomato soup.

After we were married he let me in on a secret....as a kid he hated tomatoes, unless they were on pizza! Thirty-seven years later, Phil loves tomatoes and always eats whatever I make and loves it (well, at least that's what he says).

Ingredients

    4 tomatoes - peeled, seeded and diced
    4 cups tomato juice
    14 leaves fresh basil
    1-cup almond, rice, So Delicious Coconut or goat milk or a combination
    1/2-cup earth balance or Ghee (in place of butter)
    Celtic Sea Salt and pepper to taste

Instructions

Place tomatoes and juice in a stockpot over medium heat. Simmer for 30 minutes.

Puree the tomato mixture along with the basil leaves, and return the puree to the stockpot. Place the pot over medium heat, and stir in the milk and earth balance or Ghee. Season with Celtic Sea Salt and ground white pepper. Heat, stirring until the butter is melted. Do not boil.

Phil's Famous Kitchen Sink Soup   GF, DF, NSO, HF, BF

Phil Davis (makes approximately 2 – 3 quarts of soup)
This is our most popular soup. It is a favorite from our Affordable
Healthy Eating classes and a staple at our house. We store some in
the refrigerator to eat and put some in the freezer for later.
Remove from freezer, thaw in refrigerator over night, warm on
stovetop and serve.

Ingredients
>½ head of green cabbage
>4 carrots, peeled and sliced
>1 large Yukon Gold potato, chopped
>1 large yellow sweet onion, chopped
>3 large cloves of garlic (optional), minced
>4 large leaves of kale, sliced thin
>1 small head broccoli, chopped
>2 stalks celery, chopped or sliced thin
>Celery leaves from the middle of the celery stalk
>1 14-15 oz size can organic Italian style diced
>tomatoes
>1 teaspoon dried Basil
>1 teaspoon dried red pepper
>1-2 teaspoon Celtic Sea Salt
>1-2 Tablespoons Grape seed oil (can use less or even
>none to reduce fat)
>2-3 teaspoons Organic Better than Bouillon
>vegetarian vegetable base Filtered water
>You can substitute 1-2 boxes of an organic veggie
>broth from Imagine, Pacific or Whole Foods 365
>brand (watch for MSG words) for the Better Than
>Bouillon base if you like.

**You can add any of your favorite veggies and/or add a can
of your favorite beans or a cup of cooked Quinoa for protein.

Phil's Famous Kitchen Sink Soup Instructions

Dilute Better than Bouillon in a pan of boiling filtered water, stir to dissolve. Put Grape seed oil in the bottom of your crock pot or soup kettle. Add all the veggies. With your hands, stir to coat all veggies with Grape seed oil. Stir in Celtic Sea Salt, basil and red pepper. Add the Bouillon mixture and cover with 1 inch or so of filtered water and stir well.

Cook all day, in Crock-pot or oven or at least 1 hour on the stovetop, until veggies can be pierced with a fork. This can be frozen and reheated (not in microwave) or will last about 3 days in the fridge. Only reheat enough to eat at a time, not the whole pan.

CHAPTER 15   HEALTHY VEGETARIAN PROTEINS

According to The China Study, by T. Colin Campbell, PhD. A diet of plant proteins almost entirely eliminates the possibility of cancers. Joel T Fuhrman, M.D. Eat to Live, recommends a minimum of 1 cup of beans or legumes per day.

Limit your consumption of animal proteins by eating primarily plant proteins.

BEANS – 14 GRAMS PROTEIN PER CUP

NUTS & SEEDS – 7 GRAMS PROTEIN PER 1 OUNCE SERVING

QUINOA – 9 GRAMS PROTEIN PER CUP

Weight Loss Note! Beans, Nuts and Quinoa are excellent sources of protein as long as you stick to the serving size.

They are also high calorie and high carbohydrate foods so watch your servings.

Beans (Legumes) GF, DF, NSO, HF, HP
Always buy organic canned beans as non-organic beans contain a harmful color preservative called EDTA.

Beans are the perfect protein. They are an excellent source of plant protein and very versatile. You can use them cold in salads or throw them in soups and stir fry recipes. You can buy them in cans already prepared or make them from scratch quite easily. Dr. Joel Fuhrman, in his book Eat To Live, recommends every one have 1 cup of beans per day, especially people with diabetes, high cholesterol, high blood pressure and heart disease.

The fiber to protein ratio of beans makes them a great food, even though they are high in carbohydrates, they are an unrefined carbohydrate. One cup of beans has almost half of your protein and fiber requirements for the day at 14 grams fiber and 14 grams protein and they are fat free.

Beans become a bad food when you add tons of animal fat or animal protein. Always eat and cook beans with vegetables.

If you have problems with excessive gas try taking a digestive enzyme when you eat beans and always eat raw, fresh veggies with your beans. The more often you eat beans, the fewer problems you should have with gas.

"Snuff the Fluff"
What To Do If You Have Problems Digesting Beans
- Eat beans with raw or cooked leafy greens as a side
- Don't combine beans with refined carbohydrates like breads and muffins
- Don't combine beans with animal protein

- Soak dry beans for 24 hours and rinse well

What To Do If You Have Problems Digesting Beans Continued

- Rinse canned beans well before using in a recipe
- Never add any form of salt to beans while they are cooking or they will be tough, add Celtic sea salt after the beans are cooked
- Take a digestive enzyme high in amylase and protease, such as Garden of Life Ultra Omegazyme when you eat beans.
- The more often you eat beans, the less gassy you will be over time.

How To Cook Dried Beans
Follow these Instructions for any dry bean except lentils.
Ingredients
    1 bag of any kind of dry beans
    Filtered water
    3 garlic cloves, minced
    1 sweet yellow onion, chop fine in food processor with S blade
    1 teaspoon each of dry herbs such as basil, thyme, cumin

Instructions For Cooking Beans
1st Rinse and Soak: Rinse beans well in a colander, cover with filtered water so there is about 3 inches of filtered water above the top beans and soak overnight on the counter.

2nd Rinse and Soak: Rinse beans well, cover with filtered water again so there is about 3 inches of filtered water above the top of the beans. Add garlic and onion and any spices you like.

Cook for 1-2 hours on stovetop or in 350-degree oven. Pinch beans between fingers to test for doneness; should be soft but not mushy. Drain off excess filtered water; keep any filtered water you want to use in your recipe.

How To Cook Dry Beans Continued
Do not add Celtic Sea Salt until beans are cooked or they will be hard.

You can tell the beans are cooked when you can smash them easily with a spoon.

We like to add 1-2 Tablespoons of Better Than Bouillon Organic Vegetarian Vegetable Base for richer flavor.

3 Bean Salad GF, DF, NSO, HF, HP, BF
Celeste Davis serves 4
Just like on the salad bar! Make it on your prep day and eat it with your two handfuls of greens.
Ingredients
1 can organic chick peas, rinsed and drained
1 can organic kidney beans, rinsed and drained
1 can cut green beans, rinsed and drained
½ red onion, sliced thin
1 colored bell pepper (any color), chopped
Bottled Red Wine or Italian Vinaigrette (I like Drew's Garlic Dressing) OR make the Dijon dressing

Instructions
Slice onion and pepper with slicing blade of your food processor. Mix beans and veggies. pour dressing on top and stir well. Refrigerate in a sealed container up to 3 days. Serve over mixed greens or finely sliced green cabbage

Black Bean Salsa Salad   GF, DF, NSO, HF, HP, BF

Celeste Davis adapted from a Wild Oats recipe flyer   Serves 2-3
Good for any time, however, this is a great recovery food for AFTER
your work out.   Drink 8-16 ounces of fresh veggie juice first, then 20
minutes later, eat this bean salad for muscle repair.

Salad Ingredients

¼ cup chopped green onions
1 can organic black beans, rinsed and drained
¾ cup chopped tomato (1 small tomato)
2 Tablespoons fresh Poblano or jalapeno peppers with seeds removed
1 cup chopped fresh mango or peaches
Lime wedges

Dressing Ingredients

1 teaspoon Grape seed oil
3-teaspoon lime juice (approximately the juice of 1 lime)
¼ teaspoon ground cumin
1/8 teaspoon cayenne pepper or red pepper flakes
1 Tablespoon minced green onions
1 Tablespoon chopped fresh cilantro

Instructions

Combine beans, veggies & fruit in a large bowl. Make lime dressing; pour over beans and mix gently. Chill and serve over greens with a lime wedge. Keep 3 days.

<< MAKE IT BETTER: ADD 1 CUP COOKED QUINOA FOR MORE PROTEIN.

MAKE IT QUICK: USE JACK'S SALSA (KROGER OR COSTCO) OR A FRESH PICO DE GALLO, INSTEAD OF MAKING YOUR OWN DRESSING AND ADD THE JUICE OF A WHOLE LIME AND AN AVOCADO. >>

Lentils and Brown Rice GF, DF, SF, HF, HP, BF

Celeste Davis (serves 4)
Quick, easy, packed with nutrition and very delicious!

Ingredients

> 1 cup lentils, soaked in filtered water for 1 hour
> 1 cup brown rice, soaked in filtered water for 1 hour
> 1 large yellow onion, chopped
> ½ sweet red bell pepper, chopped
> 2-3 garlic cloves, minced
> 2-3 Tablespoons Grape seed oil
> 2 cups organic veggie broth
> 2 cups filtered water
> 1 teaspoon dried basil
> 1 teaspoon cumin
> 1-teaspoon onion powder
> 1-teaspoon garlic powder
> ¼ to ½ teaspoon red chili pepper flakes (optional)
> Celtic Sea Salt to taste

Instructions

While lentils & rice are soaking sauté veggies in Grape seed oil. Add veggie broth, filtered water and seasonings. Drain lentils and brown rice. Add lentils and brown rice to pan of veggies. Bring to boil. Cover and reduce heat, cook for 30-45 minutes on the stovetop.

Basic Hummus GF, DF, SF, HF, HP, BF

Celeste Davis (makes about 3 cups)
Even people who refuse to eat "healthy food" love hummus. If you are introducing it to someone who is finicky you could call it "Bean Dip" because that is what it is.

Ingredients

> 4 garlic cloves, minced and then mashed
> 2 15-oz cans of garbanzo beans (chickpeas), drained and rinsed (or any bean you like)

Basic Hummus Ingredients Continued
½ to 2/3 cup of Tahini (roasted, not raw)
¼ to 1/3 cup freshly squeezed lemon juice
1/2 cup water
1/4 cup olive oil
1/2 teaspoon of salt
Pine nuts (toasted) and parsley (chopped) for garnish

Instructions
Using the S Blade of your food processor, combine the mashed garlic, garbanzo beans, Tahini. Start with the smaller amount of Tahini and lemon juice and add more until you reach the desired taste and smooth consistency. Slowly add lemon juice, 1/2 cup water, and olive oil.

Stop and check texture and taste. Use less lemon juice if you don't like a strong lemon flavor. Adjust your liquids to your desired thickness as all beans will use a slightly different amount of liquid. Process until smooth. Add salt, starting at a half a teaspoon, to taste.

To serve top with chopped parsley and pine nuts. Delicious as an addition to your salad, as a dip with veggies or crackers. This can be your protein for a meal.

For extra zip add a jar of roasted red pepper or a jar of sundried tomatoes or some fresh jalapeno

<< TRAVELER'S TIP! HUMMUS IS A GREAT PROTEIN TO TAKE ON A TRIP.

If you take hummus on an airplane, package it in 3 ounce see-through containers or it will be confiscated. >>

Roasted Red Pepper and Garlic Butter Bean Hummus GF, DF, NSO, HF, HP, GF

Celeste Davis Adapted from The Gilded Fork.com (makes about 3 cups)
I frequently make this hummus when catering large events, it is always a hit!

Ingredients

2 cups cooked butter beans, rinsed and drained (or any cooked beans)
1 large red pepper, roasted (or 1 jar of roasted red pepper, rinse oil off)
3 heads fresh garlic, roasted
1 cup Italian Flat parsley
2 medium green onions, cut in chunks
1 Tablespoon fresh rosemary
Juice of 3 lemons
½ teaspoon Celtic Sea Salt or to taste
1 Tablespoon tamari or Braggs Amino Acids
2 teaspoons ground cumin
½ cup expeller pressed olive oil
Dash paprika or cayenne

Instructions

Roast the pepper and the garlic (see Chapter 11). Put all in a food processor; blend until smooth, best if made a day ahead so flavors can blend. Hummus is a great way to use left-over beans of any kind. Drain liquid, rinse and use as you would a can of beans.

Black Eyed Pea Southern Style Tacos   GF, DF, NSO, HF, HP, BF

Celeste Davis Serves 2-4 A great detox food.
My grandparents loved black-eyed peas. This is my tribute to their black-eyed peas and cornbread, we enjoy this dish often.

Ingredients

½ pound of black eyed peas
1 Tablespoon organic onion powder

Southern Style Tacos Ingredients Continued

1 Tablespoon organic garlic powder
1 Teaspoon crushed red pepper flakes
4 Whole leaves of leaf lettuce (or use spelt or organic corn tortillas)
Finely shredded Cabbage
Thinly sliced yellow or green onion
Southwestern Ranch Dressing found in Chapter 11.
Sliced Avocado
Sliced Tomato

Instructions

Cook ½ pound of black-eyed peas, (soak 24 hrs, rinse and cook at 300 degrees F for 4 hours with 1 Tablespoon organic onion powder, 1 Tablespoon organic garlic powder and 1 Tablespoon organic red pepper flakes). For more information see How To Cook Dry Beans. After black-eyed peas are cooked, drain and smash slightly to a refried bean texture.

To make tacos: 1 lettuce leaf, Top with black-eyed peas, finely shredded cabbage, onion, avocado and tomato. Top with Southern Salsa.

Spicy Refried Beans GF, DF, NSO, HF, HP, BF

Celeste Davis   (serves 4 to 6)
Refried beans are a healthy, tasty and inexpensive protein. Serve with warm garlic spinach salad, Jicama salad, guacamole and pico de gallo or use for homemade bean burritos or quesadillas.

Ingredients

1 lb. soaked pinto beans
1-cup onion, chopped
1-2 garlic cloves, minced
¼ teaspoon cumin
1-2 teaspoon chili powder
1-teaspoon red pepper flakes

Spicy Refried Beans Instructions

Soak and prepare the beans for cooking, see Chapter 15, How To Cook Beans

Add remaining Ingredients.

Cook 2-3 hours at 350 degrees F (until you can smash with a spoon)

Drain and save liquid.

Smash pinto beans well, add cooking liquid as needed. Make sure smashed beans are moist; if they are too dry, they will dry out quickly when served. You can smash in food processor or with a heavy spoon or potato masher.

Save bean water in freezer and add to homemade veggie soups.

Vegetarian Bean Burgers GF, DF, NSO, HF, HP, BF

Celeste Davis
Are you hankering for a burger and fries? There's nothing like a good homemade vegan burger. Serve with all the condiments you like on a burger, use the Green Goddess Dressing, yummy! Have a side salad and oven roasted Sweet Potatoes Rosemary.

Ingredients

    2 Tablespoons Grape seed oil
    1 onion, diced
    1 clove garlic, minced
    3 green onions, diced
    1/2 teaspoon cumin
    3/4 cup diced fresh mushrooms
    1 15-ounce cans organic pinto beans, drain and rinse (or any left over beans, drain and rinse)
    1-teaspoon parsley

Vegetarian Bean Burgers Ingredients Continued
> 2 cups of organic rolled oats, ground fine in food
> processor (use gluten free if needed)
> Celtic Sea Salt and pepper to taste
> Grape seed oil for frying

Instructions

Dice onion, garlic, with S blade in food processor. Sautee onion and garlic on medium high heat in grape seed oil for 3 to 5 minutes, until onions are soft. While they are cooking, chop green onions and mushrooms. Add green onions, mushrooms and cumin and cook for another 5 minutes, until mushrooms are cooked. Set aside.

Creating The Burger

Consistency is important, just lightly mash or chop veggies, you don't want to puree them or you will have hummus instead of the firm mixture needed to form a patty.

Mash the beans with a fork or a potato masher, or process in a food processor until well mashed but not pureed.

Add the mushrooms/onion mixture to the beans and add parsley, Celtic Sea Salt and pepper. Stir until well combined. SLOWLY add ground organic rolled oats until you are able to pick the mixture up and form into patties, about the consistency of raw hamburger. Shape the mixture into patties. Heat about two tablespoons of Grape seed oil and cook each patty until the veggie burgers are done, about 3 minutes on each side.

Serve with sprouted grain buns and condiments and raw veggies to top. These will keep in the refrigerator in a sealed container for about 3 days or in the freezer for about 1 month. Reheat frozen patties in your convection oven or on a skillet after thawing.

How To Soak Nuts Seeds and Grains

Have you noticed that if you eat too many nuts you get a tummy ache? Due to modern harvesting practices and the nature in which God made them, all nuts, seeds and grains have enzyme inhibitors in them that prevent the enzymes in the food itself from being activated. This is to ensure long-term preservation. A barrel of wheat that has not been germinated can last hundreds of years. Kamut, a form of wheat, was found in the pyramids of Egypt thousands of years later and still able to produce grain. Until the food has been soaked or germinated the body cannot recognize it as food and digest it well, so you get indigestion.

Soaking the nuts, seeds and grains for 1 to 24 hours deactivates the enzyme inhibitor and releases the food enzymes, the living part of the food. The food will digest much better in your body. It also deactivates phytic acid, which prohibits the body from absorbing the calcium and magnesium in the food. Soaking times vary.

Here is the process:

Cover the food with filtered water and let it sit for the correct amount of time. At the end of the soaking time, rinse well 2 or 3 times. Put nuts on a paper towel and pat dry, then return to the refrigerator in a dry glass container. They will keep 3-5 days. Once grains are soaked they can be cooked or sprouted. Nuts, seeds and grains must be raw in order to be soaked (not roasted or toasted). Soft nuts such as cashews, pecans, walnuts and seeds like sunflower and pumpkin can be toasted after they have been soaked. 375 degrees F for approximately 10 minutes. This kills the enzymes but they are easily digested and taste better. To retain the enzymes,

How To Soak Nuts, Seeds and Grains Continued

(most important) either eat them raw, untoasted or dehydrate them in a good food dehydrator that keeps the temp under 118 degrees F.

Softer nuts like pecans and walnuts should be toasted not soaked.

You can use nut milk in place of cow's milk for all recipes.

Soaking and Toasting Times for Nuts, Seeds and Grains
GF, DF, SF, HF, HP, BF

Almonds: Soak overnight, rinse and pat dry. Keep in fridge 3-5 days

Pecans & Walnuts: Toast in oven for 10 minutes at 375.

Sunflower seeds: Soak 4 hours, rinse and pat dry. Toast in oven for 10 minutes at 375 or use untoasted.

Brown Rice: Soak 1-6 hours, and then cook as directed – you will start to love brown rice if you soak it first.

Oats, Steel Cut Oats & Oat Groats: Soak 20 minutes to 1 hour, cook as directed or sprout

Quick Cook for Steel Cut Oats or Oat Groats: Soak for 20 minutes, turn on the stove and bring the filtered water to a boil, turn off the stove and put a lid on the pan, leave overnight and they will be completely cooked and perfect in the morning. Just heat up on stove to eat, store leftovers in the fridge and use them within 2-3 days.

Wheat and Spelt: Soak 24 hours, cook or sprout

Quinoa: Soak 30 minutes, cook for 15 minutes. To sprout soak 15 minutes, put in dish on counter and they will sprout within 24 hours, then cook or use raw.

Make it Quick! Cook the entire package of Quinoa at once to save time, put cooled, cooked Quinoa in zip loc baggies and store in the freezer for up to one month.

Toasted Pecans or Walnuts GF, DF, SF, HF, HP, BF

Place any raw nuts on baking pan, bake at 450 for 3-5 minutes until toasted. Watch closely while toasting.

Homemade Almond Milk   GF, DF, NSO, HP, BF

Celeste Davis (makes about 1 quart)
This milk is fabulous; there is no comparison between homemade almond milk and what you get in a carton.

Ingredients

1 cup soaked nuts - Almonds for everyday, Cashews for sauces, soups and desserts, Macadamia for desserts
4-6 cups filtered water
Dash of Celtic Sea Salt
(for sweet milk add 2-3 Medjool dates and a dash of vanilla - for a sauce or gravy, no dates)

Instructions

Put nuts, dates, Celtic Sea Salt & filtered water in blender. Blend on high until purified. Pour through a strainer and cheese cloth several times. Refrigerate or use.

Hot Chocolate Almond Cocoa GF, DF, NSO, HP, BF

Celeste Davis (serves 1) Yummy!

Ingredients

  1-Tablespoon Raw Agave Nectar or raw local honey
  2 Tablespoons Organic Cocoa
  Dash Celtic Sea Salt
  ¼ teaspoon organic vanilla
  1-cup homemade almond milk

Instructions

Stir agave and cocoa together, add Celtic Sea Salt, stir in milk. Warm on stove top. Stir in vanilla.

Six servings of Hot Almond Cocoa

Ingredients

  ¼ cup Raw Agave Nectar
  ¼ cup organic cocoa (sift first through a strainer or sifter)
  Dash Celtic Sea Salt
  ½ cup hot filtered water
  4 cups almond milk
  ¾ teaspoon organic vanilla

Instructions

Mix agave nectar, Celtic Sea Salt and filtered water in pan, stir in almond milk, warm, and do not boil. Add vanilla and serve.

Hot Cashew Cream Gravy GF, DF, NSO, HP, BF

Inspired by The Compassionate Cook
This is delicious non-dairy gravy.   Use for biscuits and gravy or potatoes and gravy.
You can also add some Better Than Bouillon vegetarian vegetable base for richer flavor or sauté onions and garlic until very soft and add to the gravy. Basically your "milk" is from the cashews, blended with filtered water and then strained.

Ingredients

> 2 ½ cups filtered water
> ½ cup raw cashews
> 2 Tablespoons cornstarch
> 2 teaspoons onion powder
> 1-teaspoon garlic powder (less if you don't like garlic)
> ½ teaspoon Celtic Sea Salt

Instructions

Run cashews and water through blender or magic bullet until pureed well. Strain through wire mesh strainer lined with cheesecloth; this is your milk for the gravy.

Blend cornstarch, onion powder and Celtic Sea Salt with cashew milk. Cook in pan on stove top on medium, stirring constantly until thickened.

CHEF'S TIP!: AS STRANGE AS THIS RECIPE SOUNDS, IT IS FANTASTIC.

It's a great vegan gravy for mashed potatoes, to put over a bean burger or on biscuits for biscuits and gravy, give it a try!

Cashews have more protein than any other nut, 21 grams per 1/3 cup; as much protein as 8 ounces of chicken.

Sweet & Spicy Pecans   GF, DF, NSO, HF, HP, BF

Celeste Davis

These are an awesome addition to a salad, rice or quinoa dish! This will work with any nuts, cashews are especially good this way as well.

Ingredients

> 1-Tablespoon Raw Agave Nectar or raw local honey
> 1-teaspoon cinnamon
> ¼ teaspoon red chili pepper
> ¼ teaspoon Celtic Sea Salt
> 2 cups raw pecans (pecan pieces are more economical)

Instructions

Mix raw agave nectar, cinnamon, chili pepper, salt with a wire whisk. Toss pecans in agave mixture. Bake at 450 for about 5 minutes (watch them, if your oven is too hot they will burn) Bake until they are not sticking together and are dry. Cool and store in a zip loc bag.

QUINOA

How To Cook Quinoa GF, DF, SF, HF, HP

Wash Quinoa in a bowl of filtered water and "scrub" with your hands to remove the saponins. Saponins can cause a bitter flavor. Rinse well in a fine-meshed colander.

Sprout Quinoa by covering with filtered water and soak Quinoa (and all grains, even brown rice) for 30 minutes before cooking. Use 2 cups filtered water to 1 cup Quinoa, put in pan for cooking. After soaking, use same water and cook for approximately 15-20 minutes to prepare. The grain will look translucent at the end of the cooking process and the germ will pop out and look like a little tail. **For a nutty flavor, dry roast quinoa for 5 minutes in a dry skillet before cooking.

Quinoa Time Saver: I prefer to cook a 1 lb bag of Quinoa at once. After the Quinoa is cooked, put it in Zip loc brand freezer bags in one-cup amounts. When you need Quinoa for a recipe, it is already cooked! Just drop the sealed bag into a sink of hot filtered water for a few minutes to thaw.

<< *Chef's Tip!: Quinoa is a true super food. Add Quinoa to soups, salads, casseroles, and burgers; no one will know but you!*

If you feed handicapped or elderly people who must have soft and blended food, give them quinoa at each meal for intensive nutrition. >>

Cinnamon Raisin Quinoa Cereal GF, DF, NSO, HF, HP, BF

Celeste Davis (serves 2)
Gluten free comfort food, use in place of any hot cereal or oatmeal.

Ingredients
1 cup Quinoa, cooked
¼ to ½ cup Almond or Hemp Milk
1-2 teaspoons Raw Agave Nectar
1 Tablespoon organic raisins
¼ teaspoon or less cinnamon
1 teaspoon unrefined extra virgin coconut oil or organic butter
Dash Celtic Sea Salt

Instructions
Combine all in a saucepan. Simmer over low heat until thickened, stir occasionally and watch to prevent scorching.

Make up a big batch by increasing Ingredients and reheat on the stovetop each morning. Should keep refrigerated for 5-7 days.

Baked and Sprouted Quinoa GF, DF, SF, HF, HP

Toss 1 cup cooked quinoa in cookies pancakes, muffins, veggie burgers, even homemade bread to increase nutritional value and protein content.

Raw Sprouted Quinoa

Sprout Quinoa like an alfalfa sprout and eat it raw. To learn how to grow   your   own   sprouts   go   to www.thewellnessworkshop.org/recipes and click on videos; you'll find a 2-minute video called "How to grow your own sprouts".

Crunchy Quinoa GF, DF, SF, HF, HP, BF

Celeste Davis
We LOVE to sprinkle on leafy green salads or casseroles instead of croutons!

Ingredients

> 2 cups Quinoa, cooked
> 1 Tablespoon Grape seed or Extra Virgin Unrefined Coconut Oil
> 1 onion, finely chopped
> 2-3 garlic cloves, minced
> 1-teaspoon dry basil or 3-5 leaves fresh basil, chopped
> Mrs. Dash No MSG Seasoning (optional)

Instructions Preheat oven to 450 degrees F

In a cast iron or oven proof skillet: Sauté onions, in oil 2 minutes until soft, add garlic, and sauté another 2 minutes. Add Quinoa and basil, sauté another 2 minutes. Spread mixture out in skillet, bake in hot oven for about 10 minutes or until crunchy. Store in glass container or Zip loc brand bag in refrigerator or freezer. Use on leafy green salads or sprinkle on top of casseroles for crunch. Quinoa will keep refrigerated for approximately 5 days; in freezer for up to one month.

Crunchy Quinoa & Pumpkin Seed Topping GF, DF, SF, HF, HP, BF

Celeste Davis
Pumpkin seeds are anti-parasitic, it is good to eat a handful every day. This is a delicious topping for salads and veggies, we even throw some on our tacos! Use this instead of French fried onions on your cooked veggies.

Ingredients
> 1-cup raw pumpkin seeds
> Crunchy Quinoa Ingredients above

Instructions
Pulse raw pumpkin seeds with the S blade of your food processor. Add to crunchy quinoa mixture above and bake as directed above. Sprinkle on salads and veggie dishes for a savory crunch.

Alyssa's Turkey and Quinoa Casserole GF, DF, NSO, HF, HP, BF

Alyssa Mykeloff, 10 yrs old, (serves 4)
My passion and pleasure is helping families transition to a healthy lifestyle. The summer of 2009 was especially fun as I worked each week with 2 sisters, Kayla and Alyssa, ages 12 & 10 to make the meals for their family each week.
Each week we made a recipe chosen by mom, one by me and one by the girls. Then the girls and I worked together to create new recipes. This is Alyssa's favorite.

Ingredients
> 1 cup organic Quinoa
> 2 cups organic chicken broth or vegetable broth
> ½ teaspoon Celtic Sea Salt
> 1 large Vidalia or sweet onion, sliced thin
> 1 package baby Bella mushrooms, sliced
> 1 sweet red bell pepper
> 1 sweet yellow bell pepper
> 1 – 3 garlic cloves, minced
> 2 Tablespoons Grape seed oil

Alyssa's Turkey and Quinoa Casserole Continued
1 Tablespoon raw agave nectar
1 lb. ground turkey (dark meat does best) ** To make vegetarian substitute any type of cooked beans
1/3 to ½ cup Veri Teriyaki Sauce or one recipe Better Than Teriyaki Sauce in Chapter 11.

Instructions
Quinoa
Cook Quinoa in broth and Celtic Sea Salt. While quinoa is cooking, sauté onion, (red pepper optional) in oil until translucent. Add minced garlic, sauté about 2 minutes. Add raw agave nectar, simmer for about 2 minutes more.

Turkey
Cook turkey, ½ teaspoon garlic powder, ½ teaspoon onion powder, ¼ teaspoon fennel seeds (crush with spoon or grind in bullet), and mushrooms, Celtic Sea Salt and white pepper to taste, could also add basil if you like.

Combine
Mix quinoa, onion, turkey and mushrooms together with the Veri Teriyaki Sauce, serve or put in a glass dish, cover with plastic and foil and freeze for up to 2 weeks.

To Reheat Frozen Casserole
Remove from freezer and allow to sit on the counter for at least 30 minutes. Remove plastic, bake in oven for about 30 minutes at 350 degrees F until warmed through. Serve with a nice big salad.

Quinoa Chili Relleno Casserole GF, SF, HF, HP, BF

Celeste Davis serves 6
I love chili rellenos but don't want to eat the cheese that they are covered in. This recipe is a perfect substitute.

Ingredients Casserole
2 cups cooked Quinoa
1 cup chopped onion
1 cup chopped mushrooms
½ red bell pepper, chopped
1 cup Kale, chopped
2 cloves garlic, minced
Grape seed oil to sauté veggies
1-¾ teaspoons ground cumin
1-½ teaspoons dried oregano
½ teaspoon garlic powder
¼ teaspoon Celtic Sea Salt
1/8 teaspoon white pepper
2-16 ounce cans organic pinto beans in chili sauce
2 - 4 ounce cans whole green chilies, drained and cut length wise into quarters OR 6-8 roasted Poblano peppers *(I like lots of peppers)*
½ -cup raw Monterey Jack cheese

Instructions
Preheat oven to 375 degrees F. Spray or grease a 9x13 glass pan with grape seed oil. Cook Quinoa or thaw frozen Quinoa In your food processor, using the slicing blade, slice mushrooms, onion, and red bell pepper. Remove to a large skillet.

Using the S blade fine chop Kale and garlic and remove to skillet. Using shredding blade, shred cheese and set aside.

Sauté all veggies using 1-2 Tablespoons Grape seed oil until onions are translucent and veggies are tender crisp. Add Quinoa and stir in spices and chili beans.

Quinoa Chili Relleno Casserole Continued

Layer Casserole in two or three layers: (I like lots of chili peppers so I make this in 3 layers instead of two, do it to your preference. Green Chili Peppers on bottom. Top with quinoa/veggie/bean mixture. Top with some of the cheese. Add another layer of chili peppers and top with remaining cheese.

Pour Topping over, making sure it goes down the sides of the casserole (I use a knife to poke holes in the middle and push the sides of the casserole in slightly as I pour the topping over).

Ingredients For Topping

> 1/3 cup white spelt flour
> ¼ teaspoon Celtic Sea Salt
> 1 1/3 cup almond or hemp milk
> 1/8 teaspoon Tabasco sauce
> 2 eggs lightly beaten plus 2 egg whites

Instructions For Topping

Blend topping Ingredients together in magic bullet or whisk together by hand. Pour topping over casserole. Bake uncovered at 350 degrees F for one hour and 15 minutes Let stand for 5-15 minutes to set, then cut and serve.

<< *Chef's Tip!: This is a true comfort food and you may be tempted to eat more than you should.*

Cut leftovers into serving sized pieces and put the pieces in zip loc baggies. Freeze for up to one month.

When you are ready to heat, remove from baggies and place on an oven proof dish. Cover with a lid or foil and reheat 30 minutes at 350 degrees until warmed through. >>

Quinoa Pasta Salad GF, NSO, HF, HP, BF

Celeste Davis
You can use regular Quinoa or use Quinoa Pasta for this salad. Use any veggies you like or that you have on hand. This is one of Kayla's favorites.

Ingredients

1 teaspoon dried oregano
1 large clove garlic, minced
3 cups sliced cherry tomatoes
1 cucumber, chopped
1 large carrot, peeled and sliced thin
3 green onions, chopped (tops and all)
1 cup Kalamata or Greek olives, pitted and chopped
1 yellow or red pepper, sliced thin
1 handful snow peas or sugar snap peas
6 leaves fresh basil, chopped
¼ cup chopped Italian parsley
2-4 Tablespoons lemon juice
4 cups cooked Quinoa or one package Quinoa pasta spirals can be used, cook according to directions
1-cup raw feta or raw Parmesan Reggiano
Red pepper flakes as desired

Instructions

In Food Processor Use S blade to pulse (2 or 3 times) and coarse chop cucumbers, green onions, olives, basil and parsley, set aside in a large bowl. Use slicing blade to slice carrots, peppers

Combine veggies, and all ingredients in a bowl, mix gently, and allow to stand for one hour. Serve cold or at room temperature. Will keep in refrigerator for 3 days.

Gluten Free Quinoa Tabooli GF, DF, NSO, HF, HP, BF

Celeste Davis (serves 4-6)
A good choice for a side with your 2 handfuls of greens. Tabooli, a mid-eastern salad, is one of the first "new" things I tried in my first detox. Quinoa gives the texture of bulgur wheat but with good protein, a delightful new taste.
Don't have parsley or don't like parsley? Try using finely chopped spinach.

Ingredients
        2 cups quinoa, cooked
        1 sprig fresh basil
        1 bunch fresh parsley
        1/2 cup lemon juice (about 4 lemons)
        3 green onions
        1 medium organic cucumber
        1/4 cup olive oil
        2-3 springs fresh mint (2 Tablespoons chopped)
        1 garlic clove, minced
        Celtic Sea Salt and white pepper to taste
        ½ cup Greek Olives, pitted
        Leaf Lettuce Leaves

Instructions
Juice lemons

Cook Quinoa, follow instructions on package or in this book. If you have frozen quinoa, allow to thaw before adding to recipe.

<< Chef's Tip!:   To serve in a bowl, Line bowl with lettuce leaves, add Quinoa and garnish with pitted olives and a parsley sprig.

For a unique and fun appetizer or starter, fill romaine hearts with Tabooli and garnish with chopped Greek olives and some crunchy quinoa. >>

273

Quinoa Tabooli Instructions Continued
Use Food Processor. Using S Blade. First cut cucumber into chunks, put cucumber and pitted olives in food processor bowl, pulse until medium chop, remove to large bowl.

Using S Blade. Place garlic, parsley and basil, and mint, stems and all, in food processor bowl, use S Blade and pulse until fine chop, add to cucumber and olives.

Use Slicing Blade on your food processor. Slice green onions, including tops, add to other ingredients and stir.

Add Quinoa and toss gently. Add lemon juice, oil, salt and ground white pepper to taste. Store for 3 days in a sealed glass container in the refrigerator.

Quinoa Stuffed Peppers GF, NSO, HF,HP, BF

Celeste Davis
Another creation in my attempt to enjoy my favorite chili rellenos. Unlike the casserole, this uses much less cheese and is a more dramatic presentation. Makes 3 stuffed peppers, increase Quinoa and cheese to make more.

Ingredients
>   1 cup cooked Quinoa
>   1 medium tomato, chopped
>   ½ sauté on medium high heat sweet Vidalia onion, chopped
>   2 garlic cloves chopped and sauté on medium high heat with onion
>   ¼ cup fresh chopped basil or 1 Tablespoon dried basil
>   1 can organic chili beans in hot chili sauce
>   3 oz. Raw cheddar cheese (optional) shredded
>   3 organic Poblano Peppers(or your favorite kind)

Quinoa Stuffed Peppers Instructions

Cut the caps out of the peppers so they can be put back on to bake.

Sautee on medium high heat onions and garlic. Cook Quinoa, see "How To Cook Quiona". Mix all Ingredients together (sometimes I stir in some fresh salsa like Jack's). Stuff Peppers with filling. Brush peppers with small amount of Grape seed oil. Put left over Quniona mixture on top.

Bake at 375 degrees F for about 20 minutes until peppers can be easily pierced with a fork. The longer the peppers bake, the less spicy and more sweet they will be.

I put a lid on for first 15 minutes, then remove the lid to make the extra quinoa crispy.

These are fantastic to freeze, and a great "company" food. Just double the Quinoa and buy more peppers. Freeze in glass dish, cover with plastic wrap and then foil or lid.

These stuffed peppers will keep for one month in the freezer. Reheat covered with foil in the oven at 350 degrees F for about 30 minutes.

**Note: Poblano peppers are very spicy. If you prefer a milder flavor, use a bell pepper, red, yellow and orange will be sweet. You could also stuff zucchini, acorn and butternut squash or tomatoes.

CHAPTER 16   HOMEBAKED BREADS, CAKES, COOKIES, BISCUITS AND MUFFINS

NOTE: Spelt is NOT Gluten Free, however is low-gluten and may be tolerated by some people who cannot tolerate gluten.

Spelt is an ancient form of wheat that has not been changed by man. The original make up of wheat was 50% starch and 50% protein. Many altered that to make lighter, fluffier bread. Today modern wheat is 92% starch & 8% protein according to Summers Sprouted Flour research.

Spelt has a double covering which protects it from pesticides and environmental pollution. This double covering made it more expensive to bring through production; therefore it has not been changed and manipulated by man. Fortunately, spelt has retained its original make up and is still 50% starch and 50% protein.

Spelt is also a low gluten grain and contains an enzyme that helps the body to process the grain. Spelt can be used in place of any wheat flour in the exact ratio called for.

We only use Spelt flour. Many recipes call for a combination of white spelt, which has not been bleached or bromated and whole grain spelt. A combination of white and whole grain makes a lighter product; however, you can use all white or all whole grain in any recipe.

Making these recipes Gluten Free

Many of the recipes in this section can be and have been successfully made Gluten Free by using Bob's Red Mill Gluten Free All Purpose flour and 2 Tablespoons of ground Golden Flax Seed to equal spelt flour measurement. The Zucchini Chocolate Chip Muffins, Refrigerator Apple Oat Bran Muffins and Pancake recipes work very well with the above substitution. You will need to experiment with other recipes for best results.

Buttermilk Substitute GF, DF, BF

Many recipes call for Buttermilk, which is high in fat and the harmful protein, casein and if not organic, full of hormones, antibiotics, pesticides and whatever else the cow that gave the milk ate. If you do use buttermilk, use organic only.

I use a substitute of Grape Seed Veganaise, filtered water and lemon juice. This makes your muffins, moist and your pancakes tender. I use Grape seed Veganaise because it has very little soy, regular vegan mayonnaise has a great deal of soy. If you don't have Veganaise, there are other options to buttermilk that work just as well. Substitutions are below.

Veganaise Substitute: GF

1 cup buttermilk = ¼ cup Grape seed Veganaise, ¾ cup filtered water and 1 Tablespoon lemon juice or Braggs Raw Apple Cider Vinegar.

No Veganaise Substitute: GF, DF, BF

1 cup buttermilk = 1 cup alternative milk plus 1 Tablespoon lemon juice or Braggs Raw Apple Cider Vinegar.

BREAKFAST

Fluffy Spelt Pancakes   NSO, HF, BF

Celeste Davis,(serves 6)
This is a recipe for very hungry pancake eaters (12-15 medium sized pancakes) and makes A LOT of wonderful, light fluffy pancake. Be sure to use only real maple syrup. The others are just high fructose corn syrup with maple flavoring.

Ingredients
2 cups white spelt flour
1 cup whole grain spelt flour
3 teaspoons aluminum free Rumford's Aluminum Free Baking Powder
1 1/2 teaspoons aluminum free Bob's Red Mill Aluminum Free Baking Soda
2 tablespoons raw Agave Nectar
3/4 teaspoon Celtic Sea Salt
½ cup grape seed Veganaise
3 cups So Delicious coconut milk or almond milk
2 Tablespoons lemon juice or Braggs Raw Apple Cider Vinegar
3 eggs
1/3 cup unrefined extra virgin coconut oil, or Ghee, melted

Instructions
In a large bowl, combine flour, Rumford's Aluminum Free Baking Powder, Bob's Red Mill Aluminum Free Baking Soda, and Celtic Sea Salt. In a separate bowl, beat together Veganaise, coconut or almond milk, raw Agave nectar, eggs and melted coconut oil.

Heat a lightly oiled griddle or frying pan over medium high heat. You can flick filtered water across the surface and if it beads up and sizzles, it's ready!

Pour the wet mixture into the dry mixture, using a wooden spoon or fork to blend. Stir until it's just blended together. Pour or scoop the batter onto the griddle, using approximately 1/3 cup for each pancake. Watch for air bubbles and then flip and brown. Serve hot. (You can stack them on a pan in a warm oven (200-degrees F) as you are making them so the chef can enjoy pancakes with everyone.)

Special Notes
Keep the wet and dry Ingredients separate until just ready to fry. Do not over stir. Batter does not store well as if it sits, the longer the batter sits, the thinner the pancake.

IF YOU MAKE THE ENTIRE BATTER and have left overs: Option 1: Save batter for the next day, before making more pancakes, sprinkle 1-teaspoon aluminum free Rumford's Aluminum Free Baking Powder over the batter and gently stir, it will make the pancakes fluffier. Option 2: Make all the batter into pancakes, cool extras and place in Ziploc bags in freezer. To reheat, put in toaster or toaster oven. Do Not Microwave!

Light & Airy Whole Grain Spelt Waffles   NSO, HF, BF

Celeste Davis (6 servings)
Leggo your eggo, they are not very healthy for you! Make your own waffles and store in zip loc brand Baggies in the freezer, reheat in the toaster or toaster oven. Note: They won't be exactly like the frozen waffles you are used to because they don't have high fructose corn syrup and other chemicals, however, they will taste great!

Ingredients
1-1/3 cups whole grain spelt flour *I use ½ white spelt and ½ whole grain, makes lighter waffles

1 Tablespoon lemon juice or Braggs Raw Apple Cider Vinegar
½ cup Grape seed Veganaise
½ cup filtered water
¼ teaspoon Bob's Red Mill Aluminum Free Baking Soda
2 large eggs
4 Tablespoons melted coconut oil
2 Tablespoons raw Agave nectar or raw local honey
1 ½ teaspoons Rumford's Aluminum Free Baking Powder
3/4 teaspoon Celtic Sea Salt

Instructions, This Takes 2 Bowls
Bowl 1: Separate egg yolk and white (put whites in bowl 1 and yolks in bowl 2). Beat egg white until a stiff peak forms; set aside for last step

Bowl 2: Beat egg yolks well. Add raw agave nectar or raw honey, Grape seed Veganaise, and filtered water and lemon juice or apple cider vinegar.

The lemon juice or apple cider vinegar will work with the baking soda to make your waffles fluffy, don't leave it out! Beat egg yolk mixture well. Add Bob's Red Mill Aluminum Free Baking Soda. Add melted coconut oil. Add Celtic Sea Salt and spelt flour to egg yolk mixture. Beat until smooth.

Sprinkle Rumford's Aluminum Free Baking Powder lightly over the mixture and fold in quickly. Fold in stiffly beaten egg whites in into egg yolk/flour mixture. Bake in hot waffle iron. Drop onto a greased hot waffle iron according to manufacturer's directions.

Note: If you don't have Grape seed Veganaise see substitutes at beginning of Chapter 16.

Chef's Tip!

Use REAL toppings like Real Maple Syrup or real fruit toppings with Real Whipped Cream, local RAW honey or Coconut Nectar/Syrup, Real fruit spread or Fruit Compote.

Most commercial syrups are full of high fructose corn syrup, corn syrup, sugar, or corn sweetener or toxic non-sugar sweeteners.

If your children don't like real maple syrup, slowly mix the old syrup with the new until they are used to the taste of real food as opposed to high fructose corn syrup.

Roy's Fluffy Spelt Biscuits NSO, HF, BF

Roy Priszner (makes 16)
"Us southerners" love our biscuits! When I ate Roy's I had to throw out my old recipe. These are a light healthy version of the white flour and lard biscuit, same great flavor and texture. Roy makes extra, cuts them in half and freezes the halves in zip loc Baggies. When he has a "hankerin" for a biscuit he pops half in the toaster!

Ingredients
>2 cups Whole Grain Spelt Flour
>2 cups White Spelt Flour
>2 tsp Celtic Sea Salt
>6 TBSP Aluminum Free Baking Powder
>1/2 cup cold Organic Butter
>1 1/2 cups So Delicious Coconut Milk

Instructions Heat oven 450 degrees F.
In Food Processor using plastic S Blade combine dry ingredients. Cut butter in chunks and add to Food Processor bowl. Pulse a few times until looks crumbly, transfer this mixture to a large bowl.

Spelt Biscuit Instructions continued

Make a well in the center of the flour/butter mixture then add 1 1/2 cups Coconut Milk a little at a time working into the dough until dough is just tacky but not wet.

Turn out on a floured counter. Knead lightly, about 5 to 10 times. Flatten to 5/8 - 3/4 in thick round, cut with biscuit cutter. TIP (lightly grease inside of cutter so dough comes out clean)

Grease 13x9 baking pan with Grape seed oil enough to cover the bottom of the pan. Place biscuit into oil and turn over so both sides are lightly coated. Bake 12-15 minutes.

Scrumptious Spelt Flour Tortillas SF, HF, BF

Celeste Davis (makes approximately 12, 8 inch tortillas)
Once you have homemade four tortillas you'll never buy the packaged ones again! They are simple to make once you get the hang of it.
Many families make a batch or two, roll them into balls and put most of them on a cookie sheet in the freezer for about half an hour. Put the frozen balls in a baggie and take them out as needed. They will take about half an hour to thaw, then roll out as usual and cook. Fresh homemade tortillas when you want them.

Ingredients

> 1 ½ cups white spelt flour
> 1 ½ cups whole grain spelt flour
> 2 teaspoons aluminum free Rumford's Aluminum Free Baking Powder
> 1 teaspoon Celtic Sea Salt
> 4-6 Tablespoons earth balance or organic butter (cold)
> 1-¼ cups warm filtered water

Spelt Tortilla Instructions
Mixing the dough
Put dry Ingredients in your mixer or food processor.

If you are using a Food Processor: Put chunks of butter or earth balance in and pulse until flour looks like small peas.

If you are using a mixer: Use the paddle and run on high for a few minutes until flour looks like small peas. (put a towel over the top of your mixer and turn it on slowly so flour doesn't go all over the kitchen).

Food Processor or Mixer: Slowly add warm filtered water and pulse or blend on low until dough is soft and not sticky, you don't need very hot water. You should be able to pick up the dough without it sticking all over your hands, soft but not dry.

Making the Tortillas
Put dough on floured cutting board and using your hand, roll into a long snake. Cut snake into equal sized chunks and using your hand, roll each chunk into a ball. Let the dough rest for 10 minutes or longer if you like, if you are going to cook them right away. If you are not going to cook right away and want to freeze, follow Instructions at the bottom of the recipe.

Roll the tortillas
To Roll: Pat or use a rolling pin to roll each ball out into a large tortilla on a floured board. Roll it to a size just smaller than your skillet. Use a little white spelt flour to keep the dough from sticking to the rolling pin and board.

Cook the tortillas on an ungreased cast iron skillet
Heat a large cast iron skillet until you can splash filtered water on it and filtered water sizzles.

Tortillas continued. Lay rolled out tortilla on hot dry skillet, keep stove temperature about medium. Cook for a few seconds until bubbles appear then flip over to other side. Tortillas are cooked when they have brown speckles and are sort of bubbly. Put cooked tortillas in Zip loc bag or in a towel to keep warm. Zip loc bag keeps them warm and soft. Serve immediately.

To Freeze uncooked tortillas, place balls of dough on a cookie sheet and put in freeze, uncovered, for about 30 minutes, remove from freezer and place in a large zip loc bag, seal and return to freezer.

To make tortillas from frozen dough, remove as many as you want to make from freezer, place on a plate and allow to thaw for 30 minutes or until soft. When dough is thawed, follow directions for rolling and cooking tortillas.

MUFFINS AND SCONES

Organic Corn Muffins NSO, HF, BF

Celeste Davis (makes 1 dozen medium muffins)
These are great with chili and soups.

Ingredients
> ¾ cup white spelt flour
> ½ cup whole grain spelt flour
> ¾ cup organic stone ground corn meal
> 2 Tablespoons raw local honey
> 2 ½ teaspoon aluminum free Rumford's Aluminum Free Baking Powder
> ½ teaspoon aluminum free Bob's Red Mill Aluminum Free Baking Soda (Bob's Red Mill)
> 2 eggs
> ¼ cup Grape seed Veganaise
> ¾ cup filtered water
> 1 Tablespoon Braggs Raw Apple Cider Vinegar or lemon juice

Organic Corn Muffins Instructions Continued

Preheat oven to 450 degrees

You need 2 bowls

If you are making corn bread and not muffins: Put cast iron skillet in the oven at 425 while mixing your corn bread.

Mix dry Ingredients in one bowl, make a well in the center. Mix wet Ingredients in a separate bowl. Add wet Ingredients to dry all at once and stir quickly, just until mixed.

To Bake
Corn Muffins: Put approximately ¼ cup batter in each regular sized muffin cup. 1 Tablespoon for mini-muffins. Bake regular sized muffins for about 15 minutes, check at 10 minutes so you don't over bake. Bake mini muffins 6-8 minutes.

Corn Bread: Carefully remove hot cast iron skillet from oven and pour 1 tablespoon Grape seed oil or coconut oil in pan. Using a hot pad, grab the handle and swirl the oil around the pan, or use a paper towel or pastry brush to oil the bottom and sides of the skillet. Pour all of the batter into the hot skillet and bake as below.

Bake at 425 degrees F for about 25 minutes, check at 15 minutes so you don't over bake. Remove from oven, brush tops with butter. Can be frozen in Ziploc brand Baggies for about 2 weeks. To reheat, wrap in foil and put in 425-degree oven for about 15 minutes.

Serve with homemade honey butter. Make extra and freeze.

Refrigerator Apple Oat Bran Muffins DF, NSO, HF, BF

Celeste Davis (20 medium sized muffins) serving is one muffin
Forget stopping for a dangerously unhealthy Mc-sandwich or gas station biscuit. Make your muffin ahead of time and freeze or allow an extra 30 minutes in the morning to make your muffins fresh. While the muffins are baking, drink your fresh juice (and finish fixing your hair).

Bring some RAW soaked almonds or a trail mix with RAW almonds, sunflower, pumpkin seeds and organic raisins along for late morning protein.
Mix up a batch and keep batter in covered container up to 3 weeks in the fridge. Take out what you need each day for a fresh baked muffin. Healthy and delicious!

Ingredients

1 cup boiling filtered water
1 cup Eden's Organics Spelt Flakes (whole foods by the frozen bread)
1 cup organic oat bran
18 oz. (3/6 oz. cans) organic frozen organic apple juice concentrate, thawed
½ cup coconut oil, melted (extra if you are not using paper muffin cups, so you can grease your muffin tins).
2 eggs
1 ½ cups white spelt flour
1-cup whole grain spelt flour
2 ½ teaspoons aluminum free Bob's Red Mill Aluminum Free Baking Soda
½ teaspoon Celtic Sea Salt
½ cup (4 oz). Organic dried blueberries, cranberries or raisins (sweetened with apple juice, not sugar) or pulp from your carrot, apple, and lemon juice (remove apple seeds)

Refrigerator Apple Oat Bran Muffins Instructions Continued

Preheat oven to 425 degrees F

Follow these Instructions exactly and your muffins will be perfect! You need 3 bowls.

Small Bowl: Mix ½ cup spelt flakes and ½ cup oat bran together in a small bowl and pour boiling filtered water over, set aside to cool.

Large Bowl: Beat eggs, beat in coconut oil and apple juice concentrate. Add the cooled bran/spelt. Mix well

Medium Bowl: In a separate bowl, whisk together flour, Bob's Red Mill Aluminum Free Baking Soda and Celtic Sea Salt. Add dry Ingredients to wet Ingredients in large bowl then fold in remaining 2 cups of oat bran. Fold in carrot pulp, apple pulp, raisins, dried fruit or nuts, blueberries, as desired.

The batter will be somewhat thick but not really thick, it will thicken and get puffy as it rises in the refrigerator.

Refrigerate at least 1 hour "to rise" before baking.

Bake Your Muffins: Without stirring batter, fill greased muffin cups ¾ full (use butter or earth balance to grease - you don't have to grease pans or papers if you are using muffin papers.). Bake 10 minutes until risen (don't open door, look through window, if you don't have a window, just trust the time).

Lower oven temperature to 400 degrees F until muffins are browned, about another 15 minutes.

If you use mini muffin cups, reduce baking time by about half.

Refrigerator Apple Oat Bran Muffins Instructions Continued

Variations: Mix 1 Tablespoon of the carrot or apple pulp from your juice (or 1 Tablespoon grated apple or carrot), per muffin, in your muffin today! I just fill the muffin cup with the batter, drop a tablespoon of carrot or apple into the muffin batter, stir it with my finger, then bake, don't forget to lick your finger!

Note: Core apple to remove seeds if using juice pulp for baking.

To make fresh muffins daily:

Keep batter covered in fridge. Do not EVER stir it again.

Fill muffin cup, add whatever you like, carrot pulp, blueberries, shredded apples, pineapple, etc. Bake as directed above.

Spelt Chocolate Chip Zucchini Muffins DF, NSO, HF, BF

Celeste Davis (Makes 24 medium muffins or one 9x13 cake.
A Serving is one muffin or one of twenty four pieces of cake.)
Quick and easy, these fabulous, moist and chocolaty muffins have a low sugar and carbohydrate content compared to other sweet treats and the fat in the coconut oil, while saturated, is a good fat.

I make a double batch of the dry Ingredients and keep them in a sealed container in the refrigerator for up to 3 months. Then when I need a quick batch of muffins, all I have to do is assemble the other Ingredients, a real time saver!

Note: You will use 2 bowls because the way you combine the Ingredients affects the tenderness of the muffin. You also need muffin cups and a muffin pan.

Spelt Chocolate Chip Zucchini Muffins Continued

Ingredients
- 1 cup Whole grain Spelt flour
- 1 cup White Spelt flour
- 1/2 cup organic dry cocoa, sifted
- 1 3/4 teaspoons Bob's Red Mill Aluminum Free Baking Soda
- 1 teaspoon Rumford's Aluminum Free Baking Powder
- 1 teaspoon Celtic Sea Salt
- 2 medium sized organic zucchini
- 2 cups baby spinach
- ½ cup local raw honey
- ½ cup extra virgin unrefined coconut oil
- 3 large cage free organic eggs (for vegan see below)
- ¼ cup Grape seed Veganaise
- ¼ cup filtered water
- 1 Tablespoon raw apple cider vinegar
- 1-12 ounce package Enjoy Life Mini Chocolate Chips
- 1 teaspoon organic real vanilla

Instructions Preheat oven to 325 degrees F
Melt the coconut oil. Coconut oil is solid at room temperature, to quickly melt it, put a pan of water on the stovetop and bring the water to a boil. Turn the stove off and put the jar of coconut oil in the hot water, let it sit until mostly melted. Leave in hot water until ready to use.

Grate the zucchini, set aside for the final step. In your food processor, using the shredding blade, shred 2 medium sized zucchini. In the food processor bowl move the zucchini to the side so you can put in the S blade

Add the 2 cups of baby spinach and pulse chop the zucchini and spinach with S blade for a couple of pulses to make it a very fine shredded texture, **do not liquefy or pulverize**, just pulse a few times to get until finely chopped. At this point, I quickly rinse out my food processor and put it away before going to the next step.

Combine dry Ingredients in a medium sized bowl: Combine the whole grain and white spelt flour, cocoa, baking soda and baking powder and Celtic sea salt in a medium sized bowl. Use a wire whisk or fork and stir Ingredients until well blended.

Combine the wet in a large bowl: Combine honey, melted coconut oil, Grape seed Veganaise, water, eggs and real vanilla. Using a wire whisk, beat the liquid until well blended.

Put it all together: Add half the dry Ingredients to the wet Ingredients and blend well. Then stir in the following: 2 cups shredded raw zucchini. 1/2 to 1 cup Enjoy Life! brand semi-sweet chocolate chips

Add the other half of the dry Ingredients and stir until blended. Do not over beat. Pour batter into greased muffin tins or paper muffin cups, a little over half full (about ¼ to 1/3 cup if using regular sized cups. Mini cups are about 1 Tablespoon)

Bake at **325 degrees F** for 15-18 minutes. To check to see if they are done, gently push the top of one of the muffins; it should be soft but not mushy, like the Pillsbury doughboy's tummy. Allow baked muffins to cool slightly before removing from muffin pan. Cool completely on a baking rack and eat or store.

NOTE: To make as a snack cake in a 9x 13 pan, grease pan and the put batter into ban, spread evenly. Bake at 325 for about 30 minutes. To be sure it is done, put a sharp knife in middle of cake and pull out, it should come out clean (except for melted chocolate chips)

FOR VEGAN (no eggs) replace eggs in wet Ingredients with the following:

> 3 teaspoons of Ener-G brand egg replacer
> 1 Tablespoon coconut oil
> Tablespoon Grape seed Veganaise
> 2 Tablespoons filtered water.

Vegan muffins will be a little puffier and slightly drier in texture. Eliminating the eggs would also drastically reduce the fat and cholesterol content.

<< Health Tip!: A typical muffin from a "warehouse or grocery store" has a whopping 600 to 900 calories per muffin..

Compare that to all of our muffin recipes containing 120 to 240 calories per medium sized muffin. >>

RED VELVET CAKE

Red velvet cake is a bright color red when you use artificial sweeteners. Beets will give a nice red, although not vibrant red color to your cake. No one will know there are beets in the cake but you! I made this for a birthday party and everyone loved it, they thought it should be renamed OMG Cake. Even the children were asking for seconds.

Substitute 2 medium beets for spinach and zucchini.

For best results peel beets and run through juicer. Mix pulp and beet juice together and add when you would add the zucchini and spinach.

Nancy's Cranberry Spelt Scones HF, BF

Nancy Priszner (makes 10 biscuit sized scones)
This is a great recipe for company or to take on the road. You can make them more decadent by adding white or dark chocolate and your favorite nut.

Ingredients

- 2c white spelt
- 1c whole grain spelt
- 2 ½ teaspoon Bob's Red Mill aluminum free baking powder
- 1/2 teaspoon baking soda
- 6 Tablespoon cold butter
- 1/4 cup raw honey
- 1 cup Greek vanilla yogurt
- 1/4 cup sweetened or unsweetened coconut milk
- 1 1/2 cup Eden's Organic "no sugar added" dried cranberries

Instructions Preheat Oven to 375 degrees F

You need 2 bowls for this recipe.

Mix dry ingredients together: Using the S flour blade on your food processor (it is plastic), cut flour into dry ingredients by pulsing until the butter and flour have a coarse sand-like texture. Put this mixture in a large bowl.

In a separate bowl combine all the wet ingredients, blend well.

Make a well in the center of the dry ingredients, pour in the wet ingredients and mix all together using a wooden spoon and then by hand. Don't over mix.   Stir in cranberries by hand, do not over-knead the dough.

Make the scones: Pour onto a floured surface and divide dough into 3 equal portions.

293

Pat out to approximately 3/4" thick by 4"8" rectangle and cut into a desired size.

Place on a lightly greased cookie sheet arrange scones. Brush tops with coconut milk. Bake at 375 for 13-15 minutes. Best when warm, to reheat, cover with foil and reheat in oven at 400 for 10 minutes.

COOKIES & BREADS

Grandma Davis's Oatmeal Chocolate Chip Cookies NSO, HF, BF

Grandma Mary Lou Davis, adapted by Celeste Davis
(makes about 4 dozen)
We loved these cookies Grandma made for many years; a few ingredient adjustments, improve the. This recipe keeps the great taste and texture very little refined sugar and spelt flour rather than wheat flour.

Ingredients
    1 cup melted coconut oil
    1 cup melted organic butter
    ¾ cup raw local honey
    ½ cup Rapadura, Sucanat or Coconut Sugar
    4 eggs (to make vegan see below)
    1 teaspoon organic vanilla
    2 cups white spelt flour
    2 cups whole grain spelt flour
    2-teaspoon Bob's Red Mill Aluminum Free Baking Soda
    1 teaspoon Celtic Sea Salt
    2 cups organic rolled oats
    1 package Enjoy Life! Chocolate Chips

Instructions Preheat oven to 325 degrees F

Cream together in Food processor with S blade or in mixer: Melted coconut oil, softened butter, honey, and eggs, sugar vanilla. Mixture should be fluffy and well blended. It will be somewhat liquid because of the melted coconut oil and butter.

Add dry Ingredients: white and whole grain spelt flour, baking soda, and sea salt and mix by hand or with an electric mixer until well blended. Stir in oats and chocolate chips

Bake at 325 degrees F for about 8 minutes until soft and puffy. Should be soft in the middle and almost look like they are still doughy. Remove from oven and let sit on the baking pan for a few minutes, put on rack to completely cool.

Dough can be made into balls and frozen. To bake frozen cookies, put on baking pan and allow to sit for 10 minutes, bake for 10 minutes.

Vegan Cookies
The texture of vegan cookies will be somewhat puffier and drier due to the agave nectar. Substitute earth balance butter substitute for organic butter. Substitute Raw Agave Nectar for the honey. Substitute for 4 eggs and 4 Tablespoons freshly ground flax seed and 8 Tablespoons filtered water.

Harvest Pumpkin Loaf   NSO, HF, BF

Nancy Priszner and family: Makes 1 bread loaf size or 3 mini loafs or about 6 muffins. Make several batches and keep in freezer or share!
The entire Priszner Family detoxed together in the fall. Roy and Nancy and her mother, Roy's parents and his brother Randy. As Thanksgiving approached, Nancy got busy and re-created this holiday family tradition into a healthier version.

Ingredients

    1 ½ cups white spelt flour
    ¼ cup whole grain spelt
    1 teaspoon Bob's Red Mill Aluminum Free Baking Soda

1-teaspoon organic cinnamon
½ teaspoon Celtic Sea Salt
½ teaspoon organic nutmeg
¼ teaspoon organic ginger
¼ teaspoon cloves
½ cup Earth Balance or organic butter
½ cup raw local honey
2 eggs, blended
¾ cup organic canned or cooked fresh pumpkin
Your Choice of: ¾ cup Enjoy Life! Chocolate Chips, ¾ cup organic raisins or dried cranberries or cherries, ¾ cup walnuts or pecans, chopped (optional)

Instructions Preheat oven to 325 degrees F
You will need 3 bowls for this recipe

In a medium bowl Cream together butter, honey, eggs and pumpkin.

In a large bowl combine white and whole grain flour, baking soda, cinnamon, salt, nutmeg, ginger and cloves.

Mixing the Batter in a large bowl. In a separate large bowl, alternate dry Ingredients and pumpkin mixture, blend well. Stir in chocolate chips and/or dried fruit and chopped nuts.

Harvest Pumpkin Loaf Instructions continued

Baking the Bread: Turn into foil lined loaf pan.

Sprinkle chopped nuts on top if desired.

Bake at 325 degrees F. Large Loaf: 55-60 minutes, (convection 50 minutes). Small Loaves 35 minutes. Muffins 10-15 minutes.

To tell if the bread is done, use your finger to gently push the center. If it is soft but not mushy it is done.

Remove and allow to cool, remove from pans, wrap in plastic wrap and store in the refrigerator or freezer. Double wrap for freezer, can be frozen for up to one month.

YEAST BREADS

There is nothing as satisfying to me as the taste and aroma of homemade bread. The recipes in this section use yeast to rise the bread and make it soft and yummy!

Yeast is a living organism that makes bread rise and be fluffy instead of like a cracker. To grow, yeast needs warm water and a little sugar. To raise bread, yeast needs a warm, draft-free place. I use my baking oven as a simple and effective rising cabinet for all my yeast breads. You don't have to have a rising cabinet, a warm, draft free place works well. Sometimes if I am doing my laundry, I put my bread dough on top of the dryer, covered with a towel.

Yeast breads also require kneading, to form the gluten. Gluten is the protein in wheat and spelt that helps it to hold together. Kneading strengthens the gluten and helps bread stick together when you cut it as opposed to be crumbly like a muffin or a biscuit.

For a soft crust bread, brush with butter as soon as it comes out of the oven. For a crispy bread, brush with an egg wash before you bake it.

How to Start The Yeast For Breads
FOLLOW THE EXACT AMOUNTS IN YOUR RECIPE.
You need warm water, just a little too warm for your finger, about 110 degrees. You must use fresh yeast, check the date on the package to be sure it is not outdated. Yeast requires sugar to grow. I use raw honey or raw agave nectar. In a small bowl, gently stir the yeast, water and honey or agave nectar together with a spoon or fork.

297

How to Start The Yeast For Breads Continued

Set aside while you assemble all the rest of your ingredients. It takes about 10-15 minutes for the yeast to grow. When it is ready it will be fluffy, about double in size and bubbly. I love to watch yeast bubble and grow. This is what good yeast, water and agave nectar looks like after sitting for 15 minutes.

Bubbly Yeast Ready to Make Bread

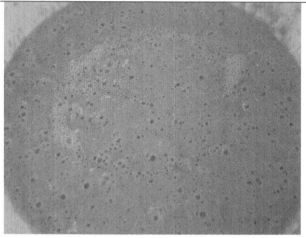

How to Knead Dough

Be sure you have a large, clean cutting board or clean counter surface with at least one cup of white spelt flour on it. Gently place your dough on the floured surface and begin to squeeze and roll the dough, like you would play dough. If it is sticky, lightly sprinkle some flour on the top of the dough and fold it in half toward you. Pick the dough up, turn it over and fold again.

How to Knead Dough Continued

When the dough is no longer sticky, you can roll it back and forth with the palm of your hand, using your whole body in a firm but gentle movement.

The dough is kneaded when it has a smooth top and can be picked up without sticking to your hands. This takes about 5-10 minutes.

How to Make A Rising Cabinet

Using your oven: Set the oven temperature for 200 degrees for 10 minutes and **then turn the oven off**.

On the stovetop, fill a pan with water and bring it to a boil.

Put the pan of hot water on the bottom rack of the oven, you may have to adjust your oven racks. Place the bowl of dough on the rack directly above the hot water, cover with a towel. Be sure the towel does not touch any oven elements or you may have to call the fire department!

Using a large food dehydrator: Set the temperature for about 115 degrees. Put a pan of hot water in the bottom of the dehydrator, put the dough in a bowl on the shelf directly above the water, and cover the bowl with a towel. Allow to rise until double in size, 30 minutes to an hour.

When we become prideful and judgmental towards others we become proud, self important and "puffed up" like yeast.

The line between discernment and judgment is often smudged by pride, disappointment and fear.

Herb Spelt Pizza Dough   DF, NSO, HF, BF

Celeste Davis makes 3 large pizza crusts
In his new book, <u>Food Rules</u>, Michael Pollan, health and food expert
says "It's Ok to eat junk food from time to time, as long as you make it
yourself". Pizza should be considered a treat, less than 1-2 times per
month. This is a great crust, the success depends on fresh yeast so buy
the bottle, not the packets and replace your bottle of yeast every
month or so. The more yeast products you make in your kitchen, the
better your yeast breads will turn out.

Making your own pizza dough is fun, taking you back to your
childhood days of playing with play dough. This recipe makes 3
regular size pizza crusts that are a medium thickness. It can also be
used to make pizza pockets or calzone. To freeze extra crust, cook,
cool and double wrap 2 of the crusts in plastic wrap and keep in the
freezer for pizza or focaccia bread.

Ingredients
1 3/4 cups warm filtered water
1 Tablespoon sugar
2 Tablespoons fresh active dry yeast
3 cups white spelt flour
3 cups whole grain spelt flour
1/4 cup Grape seed oil
1 tablespoon Celtic Sea Salt
1 tablespoon organic Italian seasoning (basil, oregano, etc)
1/2 teaspoon garlic powder or 1 teaspoon fresh minced garlic
Corn meal for bottom of crust

** you can use parchment paper and make your pizza dough directly on the parchment paper and then put on a pizza stone or baking sheet.

Herb Spelt Pizza Dough Continued

Pizza Instructions: Making the dough
Pour the warm filtered water into the mixing bowl with the sugar and the yeast. See "How to Start the Yeast", for more detailed instructions and photo.

When the yeast is active, mix in the first cup of flour. Mix in the Grape seed oil, Celtic Sea Salt, herbs and spices. Add 4 1/2 cups of flour, 1/2 cup at time, while continuing to mix the dough. The dough will be soft and may be slightly sticky at this point. Kneading dough is a great way to take out your frustration or take you back to your childhood days of play dough. Now for the fun!

See "How to Knead Dough"

Set the dough aside and let it rest while you clean and grease your bowl. Using a clean paper towel, put some olive oil in an extra large bowl and spread it over the entire inside of the bowl.

First Rising: Form the dough into a ball and place in the greased bowl. Turn the dough so it is evenly coated with the oil. Cover it to keep it away from drafts. Let rise till it has doubled in size and you can poke a hole in it with your finger.

See "How To Make A Proofing Oven"

Second Rising. When it has risen remove the dough, roll it into a large log (remember making snakes with play dough?) and cut it into 3 equal sizes for large pizzas, smaller sizes for individual pizzas, calzones or pizza pockets. Roll each portion into a smooth round ball and put on a large greased baking sheet. Put the sheet back in the warming oven or in a warm place and allow to rise again until double in size, about 30 minutes.

Herb Spelt Pizza Dough Continued
Remove everything from the oven to preheat it.

Preheat oven and pizza stone if you are using one: preheat your oven with the pizza stone in it at 475 degrees F for at least half an hour. It is vital that the stone be up to temperature before you start cooking the crust.

Shaping: Put your dough on a floured board or surface. Take each ball of dough and gently smash it into a small circle. If you are brave or experienced at making pizza dough, you can 'throw the dough" with your hands by picking it up and stretching it into a large circle, stretching it from the inside out. If you are not that brave, take your ball, smash it into a circle with your hands and roll it into a large round pizza crust with your rolling pin.

Take a fork and jab your dough (known as docking) about every inch so that the crust does not inflate like a big old pita while prebaking.

Prebaking: Turn your oven back down to 400 degrees F. Sprinkle your parchment paper, pan or pizza stone with some corn meal and slide the crust on and bake for about 10 minutes.

Top the pizza: Put on whatever you like, it's your pizza, see our ideas below.

Bake the pizza: Slide the pizza back in and bake till the toppings are cooked to the desired state. By precooking the crust, you no longer have to be concerned with making sure the crust is fully cooked.

Herb Spelt Pizza Dough Continued
For an even more flavorful crust, let it rise in the refrigerator for at least 6 hours. Remove the dough from the refrigerator 15 minutes before you are ready to roll it out.

If you pre-bake your crust you can cool it, wrap in plastic wrap and store in the freezer for 1-2 weeks. To cook, remove from freezer and let sit for about 10 minutes, put toppings on and cook on heated stone for about 20-30 minutes.

Toppings

Pizza Sauce – make your own yummy marinara or buy an organic marinara with no sugar added, no cheese, etc.

Cheese – use a raw cheese. Health food markets has a raw Monterey Jack. There are some good hard cheeses in the cheese case at Whole Foods. We love Tillamook Raw Cheese and Parmesan Reggiano. Use about 1/3 of the cheese you used in the past. The raw cheese has a lot more flavor than the conventional cheeses.

Meats – make sure you get nitrite free sausages and pepperoni, there are lots of great choices, before we went vegan my favorite was the turkey or chicken Italian sausage and some natural ground beef.

Veggies/Fruits – I love pizza w/ just tomatoes and fresh basil, make a cheese pizza and top with fresh tomatoes and basil after it comes out of the oven. Also, I love to put pineapple on it! I am getting hungry just typing this. You can put lots of different veggies, fresh, sautéed or raw on after the pizza is cooked!

West Coast Vegetarian Pizza

Marinara sauce

Red onion
Fresh Spinach cut in small ribbons with scissors
Mushrooms
Zucchini cut into strips
Raw Tillamook Cheese
Parmesan Reggiano
Fresh Basil

After it comes out of the oven top with
Fresh thin sliced tomatoes and Fresh thin sliced pineapple.

Make it with meat by adding all or one of the items below, available at Health food markets and some grocery and health food stores:

- Precooked nitrite free Italian sausage, slice in food processor using the slicing blade.
- Nitrite free pepperoni.
- Thinly sliced chicken breast sautéed in a little Grape seed oil and garlic.
- Left over roasted chicken, shredded.
- **Make it quick:** Homemade pizza is always healthier, use a flat bread pita for the crust or purchase a sprouted wheat or spelt crust from Health food markets.

Whole Grain Sprouted Spelt Bread DF, NSO, HF, BF

Celeste Davis makes 24 sandwich-sized buns or 2-3 loaves
This is a fun project.   Start approximately 3 days in advance of your
bread-making day to grow your sprouts.

Plan to be home for about 4 hours to complete the bread process, it
doesn't take that long but you do have to punch it down and knead 3
times plus your baking and mixing times. If you like to play with play
dough you will enjoy this project.

Sprouts to use: *Any grain sprouts will work; Spelt, Quinoa, Oat, and*
Rye are good choices. Learn how to sprout grains with a short video
on our website: , www.thewellnessworkshop.org

Ingredients

2-½ cups warm filtered water, 1 Tablespoon honey
or 1-2 Medjool dates in the filtered water and whir in
magic bullet

2 scant Tablespoons (2 packages) fresh active dry
yeast

½ cup Grape seed oil

½ cup honey or raw agave nectar

1-Tablespoon Celtic Sea Salt

2 cups Sprouted Grains – whole or lightly ground in
your food processor

4 cups Spelt flour (½ white spelt and ½ whole grain
spelt)

3-4 cups spelt flour (½ white and ½ whole grain
spelt)

Make a yeast sponge see "How To Start the Yeast"

To soften yeast, combine in a large bowl: 2-½ cups warm
filtered water, 1 Tablespoon honey or 1-2 Medjool dates in
the filtered water and whir in magic bullet. Add 2 scant
Tablespoons (2 packages) fresh active dry yeast and Allow
the yeast to proof (bubble) for 5 minutes.

305

Whole Grain Sprouted Spelt Bread Ingredients Continued
Stir in:
>   ½ cup Grape seed oil
>   ½ cup honey or raw agave nectar
>   1-Tablespoon Celtic Sea Salt
>   2 cups Sprouted Grains – whole or lightly ground in your food processor
>   4 cups Spelt flour (½ white spelt and ½ whole grain spelt)

Beat well
Cover with a clean dry dishtowel and let this "sponge" sit 45-60 minutes.

See "How To Make A Rising Cabinet".

After dough double in size, about 45-60 minutes, Stir down and gradually add: 3-4 cups spelt flour (½ white and ½ whole grain spelt)

Knead the dough
See "How To Knead Dough"

Turn dough onto a lightly floured surface and knead until smooth (look in a cookbook or on the internet if you don't know how to knead the dough).

Second Rising
Place dough into a greased bowl (grease with coconut oil); turn it over and around to coat the whole of the dough.

Cover and let rise until double (60-90 minutes) After this amount of time rising, the dough should be soft but firm, like the Pillsbury dough boy, if you poke it in the "tummy" it should pop back out.

Third Rising
This is where you form your dough either into loaves or sandwich buns.

Whole Grain Sprouted Spelt Bread Ingredients Continued

Knead dough down in the bowl.

If You Want To Make Loaves Of Bread

Grease 2-3 loaf pans with butter or earth balance. Divide dough into 3 equally sized pieces. Roll each piece into a big oblong ball. Place in loaf pan and allow to rise for the third time, as before for 60 minutes or until double in size. Let rise again, 60 minutes or until almost doubled

Bake The Bread Do Not Knead Again

Remove dough from proofing oven and heat oven to 375 degrees F. Bake Loaves at 375 for 35-40 minutes.

If you want to use your bread for sandwiches, do the following: Cut dough into 4 sections. Roll each section into a log. Cut the log into equal parts. Roll each part into a ball and pat into a circle about 3 inches in diameter and 1 inch thick. Put the circles on a greased baking sheet with the edges touching. Allow to rise the third time.

Bake at 375 degrees F for about 10-15 minutes.

Remove from oven and allow cooling on a rack. When cool, cut buns in half like a hamburger bun and put in Baggies in freezer.

CHAPTER 17   FAMILY FAVORITES NV

Asian Turkey Salad GF, DF, NSO, HF, HP, BF

Celeste Davis (serves 4)
A light and refreshing salad. Use on top of greens or as a sandwich filling.

Ingredients
>2 cups cooked turkey or chicken, skin removed, cut into bite-sized pieces
>4 cups cabbage or bok choy, shredded
>1 cup mushrooms, sliced
>1 cup carrots, grated
>2 tablespoons cilantro, chopped
>1 cucumber, thinly sliced
>2 celery stalks, thinly sliced
>3 green onions, thinly sliced
>1 mandarin orange or tangerine, divided into sections (can use canned)
>½ cup fresh pineapple, chopped
>½ cup chopped, toasted almonds or cashews
>½ cup Orange Ginger Dressing in Chapter 11 or your favorite organic Asian style salad dressing.
>Freshly ground white pepper and Celtic Sea Salt to taste.

Asian Turkey Salad Continued Instructions

In Your Food Processor
Slice cabbage, mushrooms, green onion, carrots, cucumber and celery with slicing blade. (It's going to all go together so just push it all through if the food processor bowl will hold it all. If not, empty food processor and continue until all is sliced). Put into a large bowl.

Switch food processor to S blade, no reason to clean out your food processor yet: Add nuts, cilantro and chicken or turkey and pulse to coarse chop. Add nuts, cilantro and chicken or turkey to your bowl of previously chopped veggies, add dressing, and toss well.

Top with green onions and oranges and pineapple, Celtic Sea Salt and pepper to taste, serve over greens. If you are not serving immediately, store veggies and meat separately, combine all with dressing just before serving. Will keep all mixed together for about 3 days but cabbage will be softer and not crunchy.

Homemade Macaroni & Cheese Southern Style SF, BF

Celeste Davis, (makes 6 to 8 servings)
This was a favorite from the 8 Simple Secrets class. This is not gluten free or dairy free however, Quinoa pasta, raw cheese, and alternative milk make it a better choice.

Ingredients
> ½ cup butter or Earth Balance
> ½ cup white Spelt flour
> ½ teaspoon Celtic Sea Salt
> ¼ teaspoon ground white pepper
> ¼ teaspoon ground red pepper
> ¼ teaspoon granulated garlic
> 4 cups So Delicious Coconut milk or Almond or Hemp milk

Homemade Macaroni & Cheese Southern Style Continued
1 8 oz. block sharp RAW Cheddar cheese, shredded
1 8 oz. block raw Monterey jack cheese, shredded
1 (16-oz) package Quinoa macaroni, cooked

Instructions
Melt earth balance in a large skillet over medium-high heat. Gradually whisk in Spelt flour until smooth; cook, whisking constantly, 2 minutes. Stir in Celtic Sea Salt, pepper and garlic. Gradually whisk in milk; cook, whisking constantly, 8 to 10 minutes or until thickened. Stir in half of raw Cheddar cheese. Stir in raw Monterey Jack cheese until smooth. Remove from heat.

Combine pasta and cheese mixture, and pour into a lightly greased 13- x 9-inch baking dish. Sprinkle with remaining sharp raw Cheddar cheese. Can also sprinkle top with some Crunchy Quinoa for crunchy top. Bake at 350° degrees F for 20 minutes (bake 15 minutes longer for a crusty top).

Homemade Turkey Sausage GF, DF, SF, HP, BF

Celeste Davis Adapted from http://www.recipezaar.com
Excellent! Use with creamy white sauce gravy for biscuits and gravy, on pizza, in spaghetti squash, or in zucchini lasagna. Freeze extra.
Instructions
> 1 lb. ground turkey (dark meat only)
> 1 – ½ teaspoon Celtic Sea Salt
> 2 teaspoons sage
> 1-teaspoon fennel seed (grind in magic bullet or crush with a spoon first)
> 1-teaspoon thyme
> ½ to 1-teaspoon red pepper flakes
> 1/4 teaspoon garlic powder
> 1/8 teaspoon ground cloves
> 1/8 teaspoon nutmeg
> 1/8 teaspoon allspice

Turkey Sausage Instructions
Use Food Processor with S blade and combine all. For best flavor let sit in fridge overnight.

Make into small patties, pan fry in Grape seed oil. Or fry up for gravy or use in recipes to replace ground beef or pork sausage. Patties can be frozen and used as needed.

West Coast Fish Tacos   GF, DF, SF, HF, HP, BF
Celeste Davis (serves 4)
Fish tacos on the west coast of the United States are fresh and fabulous, try this recipe, your family will love it!
Ingredients
¼ head Green and/or Red Cabbage, shredded

1 lb. Wild Caught Fresh White Fish – cod, snapper or halibut

1 avocado

¼ red onion

1 fresh lime

Mrs. Dash Lemon Pepper seasoning mix

Grape seed oil

Ezekiel Sprouted Grain Tortillas

Grape seed Veganaise

Lime juice and lime wedges

Pico de Gallo (or purchase Jack's Fresh Salsa from Kroger or Costco)

Guacamole

Instructions
Make cabbage slaw by shredding cabbage and red onion with the slicing blade of your food processor. Mix Grape seed Veganaise and Pico de Gallo to desired consistency, add lime juice to make the sauce thinner. Refrigerate while you cook the fish.

West Coast Fish Tacos Continued
Use: Sprouted or Spelt Tortilla, cooked fish, cabbage slaw, pico de gallo, guacamole, a sprinkle of cilantro and a wedge of fresh lime.

If you normally use sour cream try a plain, organic yogurt, we like Erivan Yogurt at Health food markets, Greek Yogurt would be my second choice.

How to Cook Perfect Fish
4 ounces of fish per person

Rub fish in Grape seed oil and place in skillet. Sprinkle fish with Mrs. Dash Lemon Pepper Seasoning and gently press seasoning into fish. Put 1 Tablespoon Grape seed oil in the bottom of your cast iron skillet. Let the fish cook undisturbed for 2-3 minutes to develop a nice crust. Cook it in batches rather than overcrowding the pan.

The best way to sauté thin fillets is to cook over medium high heat for 2-3 minutes, then turn, cook for another minute or two, then remove the pan from heat and let the residual heat cook the fish. Cook thick fillets 5-6 minutes on the first side, and then reduce heat to medium and cook for 4-5 minutes longer.

Zucchini Lasagna GF, NSO, HF, HP, BF
Celeste Davis (serves 4-6)
Delicious lasagna, without the pasta noodles. Do not use Cheese if you are on detox.
Ingredients
  Turkey Sausage or Ground Turkey recipe in Chapter 17.

  Newman's Organics Puttanesca (or your favorite) Organic Pasta Sauce

  3-4 medium sized zucchini, sliced

Zucchini Lasagna Ingredients Continued
1 small bag baby spinach
½ Vidalia onion
2 Tablespoon fresh garlic
1 Tablespoon fresh basil or 1½ teaspoon dried basil
1 raw egg
4-8 oz Raw Mozzarella, Monterey Jack or Parmesan Cheese (avoid cheese on detox)
½ teaspoon of fennel seeds

Instructions
In cast iron skillet cook sausage in some olive oil with about ½ teaspoon of fennel seeds, Celtic Sea Salt and pepper to taste.

Using the slicing blade of your food processor, slice zucchini, spread on baking sheet and lightly sprinkle with salt to remove excess liquid. Allow to sit for 10 minutes, rinse and drain.

Make Spinach Filling:
Using S blade run the following through your food processor until blended:
½ Vidalia onion
2 teaspoons fresh garlic
1 Tablespoon fresh basil or 1-½ teaspoons dried basil
1 small bag fresh baby spinach
1 raw egg

Grate Cheese (eliminate cheese if on detox)
Use the grater blade of your food processor to grate 4-8 oz. of RAW Jack style cheese or RAW Parmesan cheese. ** The less cheese the less fat and less risk of symptoms related to dairy intolerance. May also substitute rice cheese or almond cheese to make it dairy free.

Zucchini Lasagna, Layer Lasagna:
- Small amount of sauce in bottom of pan

- Layer of sliced zucchini
- Layer of spinach filling
- Layer of turkey sausage
- Light layer of pasta sauce
- Light layer of cheese (are you on detox?)
- Repeat layers, last layer should be pasta sauce and cheese

Bake in 350 oven covered for 15 minutes, remove cover and bake for 15 minutes until zucchini can be pierced easily with a fork. Let stand for 10 minutes, if necessary serve with a slotted spoon to drain any liquid from veggies.

Zucchini Crust Pizza   DF, NSO, HF, BF

Adapted by Nancy Priszner, inspired by Rachel Ray
Makes 4 personal pizza sizes or 8 small ones.
This is really good! Another find by Nancy and her mom, Gigi, to keep the family happy and eating well. Make crust and veggies ahead and keep in fridge, top and warm in convection or toaster oven.

Zucchini Crust Pizza Ingredients

1 small onion, chopped in Food Processor w/ S blade
1 clove garlic, finely chopped (1/4 teaspoon minced)
1 green pepper, sliced
1 Tablespoon chopped fresh basil or 1 teaspoon dry basil
3 cups shredded zucchini or combo of zucchini and yellow squash
½ cup cooked Quinoa
2 eggs, beaten
¼ cup white spelt flour
½ teaspoon Celtic Sea Salt
1-2 turns on a pepper grinder, white pepper
2 Tablespoons Grape seed oil

Zucchini Crust Pizza Instructions Continued

½ cup shredded raw cheddar cheese (we like Tillamook brand)
¼ cup Parmesan Reggiano (raw parmesan)

First: Put zucchini in a colander and let drain for about 30 minutes to remove excess moisture, you can press it to speed up the process.

Zucchini Crust

In a bowl, combine zucchini, quinoa, egg, flour, Celtic Sea Salt and white pepper, stir well.

In a cast iron skillet, over medium heat, splash some Grape seed oil (about 1 Tablespoon). Drop the zucchini mixture into mounds on the skillet, cook on medium for about 2 minutes per side until firm, and remove to paper towel to cool.

Topping

Sauté onions, garlic, and green pepper in a little grape seed oil until soft, fold in basil and set aside in a bowl.

Shred raw cheddar cheese and Parmesan Reggiano (raw parmesan)

Assemble

Zucchini crust
Spoonful of organic pasta sauce, your choice (read label, get low sugar)
Sautéed veggies
Cheese

Serve with a big green salad. Don't want to use cheese or on detox? Top with chopped soaked almonds or other nuts of your choice.

CHAPTER 18   DECADENT DESSERTS

On our Detox, ETC (Eat, Treat and Celebrate) plan, we enjoy one of these healthy desserts once a week! These desserts are better for you because they use good fats like coconut oil and little to no refined sugars.

Refined sugars (white, brown, raw, cane, beet, etc.) cause inflammation, which leads to pain, injury and disease. Refined sugars also reduce your immunity for up to 8 hours each time you eat something containing refined sugar. Chemical non-sugar sweeteners, although widely used are toxic to the brain, causing brain cell death and neurological damage.

You and your family will enjoy these decadent desserts.

<< Wonderful Natural Sweeteners

Stevia in liquids. Medjool Dates in place of brown sugar and in raw desserts.

To Replace White or Brown Sugar

Raw local honey, 100% Maple Syrup, Date Sugar to replace brown sugar, Rapadura, Sucanat or Coconut Sugar to replace white or brown sugar >>

Choconut Pie Filling GF, DF, NSO, BF

Celeste Davis (one 9-inch pie)
This is a delicious creamy pie, without the health hazards of cow's
milk. You can use it as a chocolate cream pie filling.
At our Whole Foods cooking class our Almond Joy pie crust came out
of the oven looking like a chocolate Frisbee, we broke it into pieces,
layered it with this pie filling and topped with a dollop of whipped
cream, everyone loved it!
Make piecrust with spelt flour or use the Almond Joy Crust.
Make filling, fill piecrust, and cover with wax paper, sprinkle top with
shaved chocolate or coconut and refrigerate.

Ingredients
>   6 Tablespoons organic Corn Starch
>   ½ cup organic unsweetened powdered Dutch Cocoa
>   4 Tablespoons filtered water
>   ½ cup Raw Agave Nectar
>   2-4 Tablespoons Raw organic Tahini (to taste)
>   2 teaspoons organic real Vanilla
>   1/8 – ¼ teaspoons Celtic Sea Salt
>   2 cups of SO Delicious Unsweetened Coconut Milk
>   1 cup of So Delicious Coconut Creamer

Instructions
Make the chocolate mixture:

In a medium glass dish mix with a whisk until smooth and
well blended

>   6 Tablespoons organic Corn Starch
>   ½ cup organic unsweetened powdered Dutch Cocoa

Add 4 Tablespoons COLD filtered water and whisk until it
makes a smooth paste. (you could also do this in your magic
bullet).

Choconut Pie Filling Instructions continued
Add And Whisk In Until Smooth:

> ½ cup raw honey or coconut syrup
> 2-4 Tablespoons Raw organic Tahini (to taste)
> 2 teaspoons organic real Vanilla
> 1/8 – ¼ teaspoons Celtic Sea Salt

In a medium saucepan heat until warm: 2 cups of SO Delicious Unsweetened Coconut Milk and 1 cup of So Delicious Coconut Creamer. Slowly stir Chocolate mixture into milk with a whisk. Stir constantly over medium heat until mixture bubbles and thickens.

Pour into finished pie shell (use the Almond Joy Pie Shell Below). Cover top with waxed paper, refrigerate

To Serve
Remove waxed paper, Cover top of pie with Real Whip Cream, chocolate shavings and some flaked coconut Enjoy!

Almond Joy Pie Crust GF, DF, NSO

Celeste Davis, Roy & Nancy Priszner (makes one 9 inch pie crust)
This is a quick and easy pre-baked crust, can be made up to 2 days in advance, refrigerate and cover w/ plastic wrap. You can also break it up after it is baked and cooled and use as a topping or layer for puddings and cakes.
Ingredients:

> 2 oz. organic semi-sweet chocolate, melted in oven, stove top or over filtered water (not microwave)
> 2 Tablespoons Earth Balance
> 2 Tablespoons Raw Agave Nectar
> 1 ½ cups unsweetened organic shredded coconut
> Crushed Raw Almonds and Pinch of Celtic Sea Salt

Almond Joy Pie Crust Instructions

Grease pie plate well with butter or earth balance and sprinkle bottom and sides with ¼ cup crushed almonds.

Using a double boiler, combine chocolate, earth balance and raw agave nectar or raw honey and a pinch of Celtic sea salt. Reserve coconut and crushed raw almonds.

Melt chocolate mixture, be careful not to allow water to splash in. Do not over cook, just until it is melted and smooth. Add rest of crushed almonds and coconut to chocolate mixture, stir quickly, you may need to mix it with your hands (no licking fingers until your pie crust is finished!) Pat into bottom and sides of pie pan.

Bake at 350 degrees F, about 20 minutes, until firm but not dark.

After the shell is baked it may be a disk in the bottom of a pie pan. Sprinkle crushed raw almonds over the top and using a cup, gently smash the disk from the center out to make it go up the sides of the pie pan. Cover with plastic wrap and put another pie pan on top to cool and retain the pie shape.

Cool, remove plastic wrap and fill w/ chocolate pie filling. This would also be delicious with a coconut cream pie filling.

Spelt Pie Crust SF, BF

Celeste Davis (makes two 9 inch pie crusts)

Ingredients

- 2 cups white spelt flour
- 1 teaspoon finely ground Celtic Sea Salt
- 1/3 cup cold organic unsalted butter, cut in pieces
- 1/3 cup cold organic Earth Balance shortening, cut in pieces
- 5-7 tablespoons ice cold filtered water
- 2 teaspoons Braggs Raw Apple Cider Vinegar or lemon juice

Put flour and Celtic Sea Salt in food processor with S blade. Add butter and earth balance and PULSE until the flour/butter looks like small peas.

Mix ice water and vinegar or lemon juice (makes the crust more tender). Slowly pour the liquid into the food processor as you pulse until it all comes together in a ball.

Move dough to floured board, pat and then roll out to a little larger than your pie pan. Gently fold in half and put in pie pan to cover one half of the pan, unfold to fill the pan.

Gently fit crust into pan and trim the edges so they are even. Crimp edges.

To bake empty crust, prick crust with fork and bake at 350 degrees F for about 18 minutes, until golden.

To bake with a filling, follow the directions for your filling.

To freeze unbaked shell, prick well and stack pie shells with parchment paper in between each shell. Seal well with plastic wrap. Freeze up to 6 weeks.

To bake frozen, unbaked shell, put in 475 degree F oven until golden.

Fresh Whipped Cream   GF, NSO

Celeste Davis (makes 1 ½ cups)
Whipped Cream is easy to make and delicious. Don't buy the poison frozen non-dairy topping, make your own real whipped cream!

Ingredients
> 1 cup organic whipping cream or heavy cream, very cold (don't freeze or it will turn to butter, trust me)
> 1-2 Tablespoons Raw Agave Nectar, also cold
> Dash of Celtic Sea Salt

Instructions
Put bowl and beaters in the freezer to chill (15 minutes). In the chilled bowl, whip cream and Celtic Sea Salt on high until soft peaks form.

Add raw agave nectar and/or 2 drops of Stevia (to taste) and whip until stiff peaks form.

Whip Cream Frosting GF, NSO

Celeste Davis (frosts one cake)
Use this on the Gigi's Garden Chocolate Cake or any of your favorite cakes. It's light and luscious!

Ingredients
> 1 8 ounce package organic cream cheese, softened
> ¼ cup raw agave nectar, cold
> 1 teaspoon organic vanilla extract
> 2 cups organic heavy whipping cream, VERY COLD

Instructions
Put large bowl and beaters in freezer to chill. Using chilled bowl and beaters, whip cream cheese, raw agave nectar, and vanilla in the large, cold mixing bowl until smooth. Keep mixer running and slowly pour in whipping cream. Whip until it makes a stiff peak, scraping sides and bottom as needed. If you whip too long, it will become butter. Frost cake as desired.

Chocolate Ganache GF, NSO

Celeste Davis
This is a rich chocolate pudding type filling for cakes and cream puffs. Use with Gigi's Garden Chocolate Cake or layer with whip-cream and fruit for a beautiful parfait.

THIS RECIPE MUST BE MADE AHEAD AND CHILLED FOR 2 HOURS BEFORE FINISHING AND USING.

Ingredients
    1 package of Enjoy Life Chocolate Chips
    1 ½ cups organic heavy whipping cream
    1 Tablespoon flavored liqueur (orange or cherry would be best) or almond or peppermint extract

Instructions
Step One: In a double boiler, melt chocolate chips and whip cream, stirring constantly. Don't let any filtered water splash into the chocolate. Stir in liqueur or extract, blend well.

CHILL FOR 2 HOURS, PUT MIXER BEATERS IN THE FREEZER WHILE CHILLING.

Step Two: Remove from refrigerator and beat with cold beaters on high for 20-30 seconds until soft peaks form.

Use immediately as cake filling or in a parfait with whipped cream and crumbled Choconut pie crust and/or fresh berries.

Gigi's Garden Chocolate Cake NSO, HF, BF

Celeste Davis (makes two 8 inch round cakes)
This is a decadent, visually stunning and yet somewhat healthy chocolate cake. No one will ever know there is zucchini hidden inside! Moist, beautiful and decadent without the refined sugars.
It's not difficult but it does have several steps, it's not something you can just "whip up". Make it quick with Individual Garden Chocolate Cakes.

Steps To Make Cake

1. Make 1 recipe of Spelt Chocolate Chip Zucchini Muffins and divide batter into 2 round cake pans (I like to use spring form pans.) Grease each pan and put a circle of parchment paper in the bottom of each pan.

2. Make 1 recipe of Chocolate Ganache Filling.

3. Make 2 recipes of Whipped Cream Frosting.

4. Assemble, (the cake looks beautiful on a glass footed cake platter).

- 1 cake round on a cake platter
- Put ½ Ganache filling on top of cake round so it is the same thickness as the cake round, smooth to the edge so it is even all the way across.
- Refrigerate so Ganache filling becomes firm.
- Put ½ Whipped Cream Cheese Frosting on top of Ganache filling gently spread over Ganache filling.
- Gently put second cake round on top of Whipped Cream Cheese Frosting.
- Smooth out filling and whip cream frosting that may be poking out of the sides of the cake with a straight edge spatula or knife.
- Chill for 2 to 24 hours.

Individual Gigi's Garden Chocolate Cakes   NSO, HF, BF

Celeste Davis (makes 24 muffin type cakes)
See the Garden Chocolate Cake recipe for Ingredients and Instructions, this is a different and somewhat simpler version.

Ingredients

1 Chocolate Chip Zucchini Muffin per person
1 recipe Chocolate Ganache filling, recipe
1 recipe Whipped Cream Cheese Frosting, recipe

Individual Garden Chocolate Cakes continued
Assemble one per person on a dessert plate
- One zucchini chocolate chip muffin cut in half, put the bottom half in the middle of the plate.
- Top the bottom half of the muffin with 1-2 Tablespoons Chocolate Ganache Filling, try to make the Ganache fit on the muffin without spilling over.
- Refrigerate for up to half an hour. Remove from refrigerator, put 1-2 Tablespoons Whipped Cream Cheese Frosting on top of pudding, and put muffin top on the frosting.
- Just before serving, top with a dollop of organic whipped cream and a maraschino cherry or a few fresh raspberries and a sprig of fresh mint.
- Serve at room temperature.

Nacho Strawberries NSO, HF

Celeste Davis inspired by Mexican Restaurants!
(makes 6 serving is 1 wedge, 1 tortilla makes 6 wedges)
This simple dessert is a great end to a Mexican fiesta!
Ingredients
1 Spelt flour tortilla
6 fresh strawberries (can also use frozen)
1-2 Tablespoons raw honey or coconut syrup
1 pint fresh whipping cream
2 Tablespoons melted Earth Balance vegan buttery stick or unsalted butter (optional)
1-Tablespoon raw honey or coconut syrup
1 teaspoon Organic cinnamon

Strawberry Nacho Instructions
Prepare tortillas (can be done ahead of time)
Make or buy spelt flour tortillas.

Brush with melted butter. (optional) Sprinkle with sugar & cinnamon (optional). Cut into pie shaped wedges. Bake at 350 for 10 minutes or until crisp, not brown.

Prepare strawberries (can be done ahead of time)

Coarse chop strawberries in food processor. Add 1-2 Tablespoons raw agave nectar or local raw honey, stir well, consistency should be thick, not runny.

Assemble (must be done just before serving)
- 1 tortilla wedge
- 1 small spoonful strawberries
- 1 small dollop whip cream
- Sprinkle with cinnamon

FROZEN DESSERTS

Homemade Ice Cream GF, NSO, BF

Celeste Davis (approximately one quart ice cream)
Make in your Cuisinart Ice Cream Maker, no mess from salt, turning a crank or chopping ice. We keep our Cuisinart ice cream tub in the freezer at all times so we can use it when we get the urge for some great ice cream. It just takes about 25 minutes, less time than getting in the car and driving to the ice cream shop.

Ingredients
1 ½ cups So Delicious Coconut Milk, unsweetened
(can also use cow's, hemp or almond milk)
1 cup So Delicious Coconut Creamer (or other cream or creamer)
½ cup Raw Agave Nectar
1-2 teaspoon organic pure vanilla

Homemade Ice Cream Instructions

Use a mixer or whisk to mix the Ingredients well. Put in freezer for 15-30 minutes to chill.

Follow Instructions for your ice cream maker.

Add fruit, chocolate, chocolate chips, almond butter, nuts, whatever you like before you freeze the ice cream or enjoy over fresh fruit!

Homemade Popsicles GF, DF, NSO

Celeste Davis (serves: 4)
These are quick, easy and delicious, as well as being healthy! Let the kids help make a batch each week and keep them on hand all summer long.

Ingredients

> 2 cups cut-up summer fruit (strawberries, peaches, watermelon, etc.)
> 1 tablespoon Agave Nectar or Raw Honey
> 1 teaspoon fresh lemon juice

Instructions

Place the fruit in a blender or magic bullet. Cover and blend until smooth.   Add 1-2 tablespoons filtered water, if necessary to thin consistency. Add raw agave nectar and lemon juice.   Cover and blend until well mixed.

Pour into 4 oz. ice-pop molds or paper cups. Insert sticks or wooden or plastic spoons. Freeze until solid.

The least messy way is to put paper cups into a muffin tin, fill the cups about ¾ full and then put your "sticks" in and freeze.

If sticks tend to fall over, use some tape and create a grid across the tops of the cups with the tape to hold the spoons or sticks upright.

More Popsicle Ideas
To make creamy add So Delicious Coconut Creamer or Erivan or Oikos Greek Yogurt, adjust flavors to taste.

Wallyade Juice is also excellent for popsicles!

Monkey Bites GF, NSO, BF

Celeste Davis (serves 2)
Yummy & Quick! This is a spur of the moment, :I'm hungry for something chocolate and cold type of treat. To keep frozen bananas in the freezer, peel ripe banana, put in baggie and freeze.

Ingredients
> 2 frozen bananas
> 2 Tablespoons Enjoy Life Chocolate Chips
> 2 Tablespoons Raw Almond Butter
> 1 teaspoon unrefined extra virgin coconut oil

Instructions
The hardest part is melting the chocolate. Don't use a microwave or you will turn into a frog!

Melt chocolate chips, almond butter and oil in a pan over a double boiler. Do not allow water to splash into pan or chocolate will separate.

If you don't have a double boiler: Put water in a saucepan and bring it to a boil. Put chocolate chips, almond butter and coconut oil in a smaller pan. Put smaller saucepan over pan with the boiling filtered water.

Stir Ingredients until melted. Don't allow water to splash into pan with chocolate or chocolate will separate.

Remove bananas from freezer and slice frozen bananas into thick bite sized slices, put in 2 bowls (one for each person)

Drizzle chocolate mixture over bananas and allow to rest for a minute or two until chocolate hardens on banana. Enjoy!

Nutty Buddy Almond Butter Balls GF, DF, NSO, HP, BF

Celeste Davis (makes 12 balls) Serving size is 1-2 balls PER DAY
My version of an ever popular raw almond treat!

Ingredients
- 1/2 cup raw almond butter
- 1/2 cup soaked sunflower seeds
- 1/2 cup organic raisins
- 1-2 Tablespoons raw local honey

Instructions

Using your Food Processor S Blade: Grind sunflower seeds to smooth. Add almond butter and raw agave nectar, blend well. Add raisins and pulse until blended. Roll into 2 inch balls. Can roll in coconut if you like!

Baked Apples GF, DF, NSO, HF, BF

Celeste Davis (serves 8) Count as a fruit on detox

Ingredients
- 4 cooking apples (granny smith)
- 8 Tablespoons raisins
- Cinnamon to taste
- Splash of Grape seed or coconut oil
- Splash of pure vanilla extract

Instructions

Cut apples in half, core out middle. Drizzle apples with oil and sprinkle with cinnamon and vanilla. Fill middle of apple with raisins. Bake 350 degrees F for 45 minutes You can substitute blueberries or cranberries for raisins, just put in the last 15 minutes

Baked Apples, Make Them Decadent! (after detox)

1 baked apple, add 1 small scoop So Delicious Coconut Vanilla Ice Cream (most groceries carry this). Drizzle with 1 teaspoon raw honey, dip knife in honey and drizzle over ice cream, the honey hardens like caramel. Sprinkle with 1/2 teaspoon chopped pecans or walnuts.

Phil's Fruity Sorbet GF, DF, NSO

Phil Davis (makes 4 half-cup servings)
*You can have this every day on detox, **count as one of your fruits**.*

Ingredients

2-3 frozen bananas (freeze without peel)
1 cup of any type of Frozen fruit you enjoy
(blueberries, strawberries, raspberries, etc)
Raw Agave Nectar for sweetness as needed

Instructions

Peel fresh bananas, the riper the better, and put in Ziploc Baggies. Store in freezer. They will keep for about one month.

Using Your Champion Or Green Star Juicer:

Feed frozen bananas and fruit through juicer with blank screen attachment in place, OR place in food processor and blend until super smooth.

Raw Peach Cobbler GF, DF, NSO, HF, HP, BF

Celeste Davis (makes an 8x8 pan)
This is to die for! Peaches do not turn brown and it will keep at least 3 days in the refrigerator.

Fruit Filling

7 large peaches, remove skins and pits
½ teaspoon cinnamon
1 Tablespoon unrefined coconut oil
Dash Celtic sea salt

Raw Peach Cobbler continued
Filling Instructions
Put 3 skinned and pitted peaches in your magic bullet or food processor and puree. Add cinnamon and coconut oil and salt and blend well. It should resemble baby food. Thin slice remaining skinned and pitted peaches. Pour pureed peaches over sliced peaches and stir until sliced peaches are well covered.

Crumb Topping
> ½ cup pecans
> ½ cup cashews
> ¼ cup toasted organic oatmeal flakes
> 1 cup Medjool dates, pitted
> 2 Tablespoons unrefined coconut oil
> ½ teaspoon cinnamon
> 1 teaspoon almond or vanilla extract

In Food Processor, using S blade, pulse dates until finely chopped. Add nuts, oatmeal, oil, cinnamon and extract and pulse until well blended but coarse (not a paste).

Put fruit filling in pan. Crumble topping over filling. Press topping down lightly over peaches. Cover and refrigerate.

These are products we have used. We do not endorse these products or their manufacturers or receive compensation for using or listing them.

CHAPTER 19
RESOURCES AND READING

ON LINE FOOD SOURCES AS OF 6/2010

(also available at Health food marketss, health food & grocery stores)

Organic, Non-GMO Corn Chips
http://salsaxochitl.elsstore.com/view/category/1672-chips/

ShaSha Spelt Products
http://www.shashabread.com/product/36/format/4

Enjoy Life Chocolate Chips and other Gluten Free Products
http://www.enjoylifefoods.com/where_to_buy/store_locator_grocery.php

Grape seed Oil
http://www.spectrumorganics.com/?id=6

Coconut Oil
http://www.wildernessfamilynaturals.com/mm5/merchant.mvc?

Quinoa
http://www.nutsonline.com/cookingbaking/grains/quinoa/white-new?gclid=CMv01dac358CFRq1sgodxifOHg

Raw Agave Nectar

http://www.wildernessfamilynaturals.com/mm5/merchant.mvc?

Raw Almond Butter

http://www.wildernessfamilynaturals.com/mm5/merchant.mvc?

Stevia

http://www.wildernessfamilynaturals.com/mm5/merchant.mvc?

Celtic Sea Salt

http://www.celticseasalt.com/

Grape seed Veganaise

http://www.followyourheart.com/products.php?id=20

BOOKS WE READ AND TRUST

These are authors we trust who have proven track records in Natural Health, read them several times to absorb the truth.

BOOKS ABOUT FOODS THAT HEAL

Enzyme Nutrition, Dr. Edward Howell, Avery, 1985

The Healing Power of Enzymes, Dr. DicQie Fuller, Forbes, 1998, 2005

Encyclopedia of Healing Foods, Michael Murray, N.D., Atria, 2005

Prescription for Nutritional Healing, Phyllis A. Balch, CNC, James F. Balch, M.D., Avery, 2000

Raw Juices Can Save Your Life, Sandra Cabot, M.D., WHAS, 2001

Hallelujah Diet, George Malkamus, Destiny Image Publishers, Inc. ISBN 13:978-0-7684-2321-1, 2006

Eat To Live, Joel Fuhrman, M.D., Little, Brown and Company, 2003

Thrive, Brendan Brazier, Penguin, 2007

Eat Right 4 Your Type, Dr. Peter J. D'Adamo. Berkley Books 1999

Fell's Official Know-It-All Guide, Health & Wellness, Dr. M. Ted Morter, Jr. M.A. ISBN # 0-88391-022-5, Fredrick Fell Publishers, 2000

BOOKS ABOUT WHAT'S IN YOUR FOOD

The China Study, T. Colin Campbell, PhD, & Thomas Campbell II, Benbella Books, 2006

The Un Healthy Truth, Robyn O'Brien, Broadway Books, 2009

Mad Cowboy, Howard F. Lyman, Touchstone, 1998

Suicide by Sugar, Nancy Appleton, PhD, Square One Publishers, ISBN 978-0-7570-0306-6, Square One Publishers, 2009

Food Inc, The Movie order on-line, http://www.foodincmovie.com/, 2009

Are Your Kids Running On Empty?, Ellen Briggs, Sally Byrd, N.D., Many Hands Publishing, 2004

BOOKS TO HELP CHANGE OTHER AREAS OF YOUR LIFE

Winning After Losing, Stacey Halprin, Warner Wellness 2007

Today Matters, John C. Maxwell, Center Street, 2004

Total Forgiveness, R.T. Kendall, Strang Communications, 2002, 2007

The Holy Bible, Thompson Chain-Reference Study Bible, New King James Version, Publishers, B.B. Kirkbride Bible Co. Inc., ISBN 13: 978-0-8870-7008-2

There are many types of natural healing therapies available today. Phil and I are committed to only submit our body to the hands and mind of someone who is a follower of Jesus Christ.

The scripture is very clear that we should be careful about the "laying on of hands". There are many health care practitioners who, while they are gifted in healing and proficient in knowledge and skill, do not follow Jesus Christ but other religious philosophies. This cannot help but be reflected in the perspective in which they treat their patients. There are other practitioners who are devoted to new age and eastern religious philosophies and encourage their patients and clients to follow these for healing.

This is America and all are free to follow whomever they choose, however, we believe it imperative to get our advice from those who have a biblical perspective and are wholly committed to a personal relationship with The Healer who took 39 beatings on His back to provide healing for the 39 major diseases in this world, Jesus Christ.

If you share our value in this area, following this philosophy requires some homework on your part. Many times checking a website will give you clues to a practitioner's philosophy. Pray and ask the Holy Spirit to direct you to the right person and always use discernment, not out of fear of man but out of respect for the wisdom of the God who created your body.

We have links on our website for practitioners who follow Jesus Christ and offer services in Medical Treatment, Chiropractic Care, Massage Therapy, Rain Drop Massage, Young Living Oils, and Colon Hydro Therapy. We have confidence in supplements made by Standard Process, Transformation Enzymes, Garden of Life, Some Nutri-West and some Jay Robb, Udo's Choice.

www.thewellnessworkshop.org

Medical Doctors with a well-balanced approach:

Be sure to visit our website

http://thewellnessworkshop.org

Check out our web-based 4 month coaching program, My Busy Healthy Life with special editions for women and men on our website. Weekly instructions walk you step by step to the life you've always wanted.

Sign up on the website for the RSS feed on our blog for regular updates on healthy living and more Wonderfully Well recipes.

We are available to speak to your church, business or community group. For more information go to the Church & Corporate Wellness Page on our blog.

We love to share our Wonderfully Well message in a fun and relevant way with groups of all ages and all walks of life.

Call Celeste at 615-975-0186 for booking information.

We are able to coach individuals and families from time to time as our schedule allows. For more information call Celeste at 615-975-0186.

The Wellness Workshop

615-975-0186

www.thewellnessworkshop.org

What to buy organic and Ingredients to avoid.

Easy Prepared Food Rule: If the package lists more than 5 ingredients that are not real food (i.e.: broccoli, milk, etc.) or has words that say "glutamate, corn" or chemical words, don't buy it, the food contains toxic ingredients.

Cut this out, fold in the middle, laminate it at Staples or Kinkos and keep it in your wallet or purse, refer to this list when shopping.

Many companies are advertising "No High Fructose Corn Syrup" however; when you read the ingredients you will many times see **maltodextrin, which is corn sugar or syrup.

Apples	Peaches	Spinach
Grapes	Pears	All Lettuces
Celery	Peppers	Spring Mix
Cherries	Potatoes	**All Meats**
Corn	Raspberries	**Dairy Products**
		ORGANIC ONLY

We Avoid These Ingredients: Milk/Dairy: rBGH, BHT, BHA. **Meat:** Nitrites, Nitrates, Antibiotics, Hormones. **Sweeteners:** Sugar, Cane Sugar, Cane Syrup, High Fructose Corn Syrup, Corn Syrup, Maltodextrin, **Non-Sugar Sweeteners:** Splenda, Sucralose, Equal, NutraSweet, Sweet n Low, Aspartame, Truvia, Xylitol, Malitol. **Packaged, Canned or Frozen Foods:** Corn, Cottonseed, Canola and Soybean Oils, Blue, Yellow, Red Dyes, Trans Fats, MSG, Hydrolyzed & Autolyzed Yeast, BPA

343